Commandments of Weight Loss

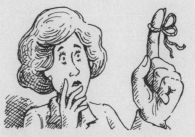

8. Thou shalt be patient but not forgetful.

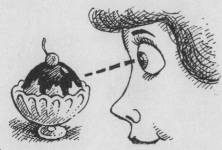

5. Thou shalt eat not when thine eye lusteth, but when thy stomach requireth sustenance.

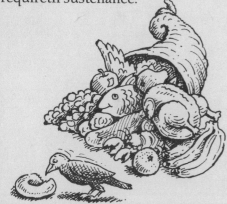

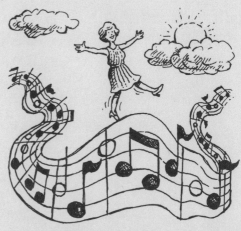

9. Thou shalt take delight in every good friend and good song, in every good walk and good day, for to enjoy them more is why these commandments are given unto thee.

6. Thou shalt sup chiefly on the fruits of the earth, the grains and vegetables thereof; on the fowl of the air and the fish of the seven seas, whence donuts cometh not.

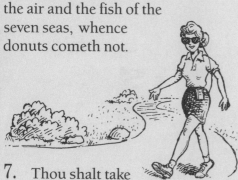

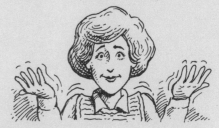

10. Thou shalt not knit thy brow if thou transgress a commandment, but forgive thyself, for it is written, nine out of ten is not bad.

7. Thou shalt take exercise daily, for why else hast thou sinew and bone, legs and sneakers?

Lose Weight Naturally

NEW, Revised Edition

Lose Weight Naturally

The No-Diet, No-Willpower Method of Successful Weight Loss

NEW, Revised Edition

By Mark Bricklin

Editor,
PREVENTION Magazine

Rodale Press, Emmaus, Pennsylvania

Copyright © 1989 by Rodale Press, Inc.

Printed in the United States of America

Book design by Acey Lee

Library of Congress Cataloging-in-Publication Data

Bricklin, Mark.
    Lose weight naturally : the no-diet, no-willpower method of successful weight loss / by Mark Bricklin. — New, rev. ed.
        p.   cm.
    Includes index.
    ISBN 0-87857-765-3   hardcover
    1. Reducing diets.   2. Reducing.   I. Title.
RM222.2.B775   1989
613.2′5—dc19   88-28335
                                                                                              CIP

Distributed in the book trade by St. Martin's Press

2   4   6   8   10   9   7   5   3   hardcover

For Rita

Contents

Contents

Acknowledgments

Special contributions to this new, revised edition were made by Jennifer Whitlock, executive editor of the *Lose Weight Naturally Newsletter*. I am also grateful for the contributions of the staff of *Prevention* magazine and all Rodale health publications.

PART

I

The Mindstyle of Lifetime Slenderness

1

Now for Something Completely New

The first question everyone asks about a new diet plan is "How is this diet different? Why is it going to succeed when all the other diets I've tried failed?"

These are perfectly legitimate questions, and I want to answer them immediately. But I'm going to do that by making eight statements about weight reduction and asking you to read each of them and decide which are true and which are false. *Please think carefully before answering.*

1. My problem is that I need to lose weight—20 or 30 or 50 or however many pounds.   T   F
2. When you're following a diet, there's no substitute for willpower.   T   F
3. To follow a diet successfully, you need a special eating plan and special low-calorie meals. At least, they're a big help.   T   F
4. Three pounds a week is about the minimum loss that a good diet should produce.   T   F

5. In general, it's a good idea for the reducer to avoid
   such starchy, high-carbohydrate foods as bread,
   potatoes, beans, rice and spaghetti.   T   F
6. Fact: To burn up the calories in one piece of pie a
   la mode, you would have to do 50 push-ups, 100
   deep knee bends and 200 sit-ups, and then run
   around the block half a dozen times! So exercise
   isn't really that important in reducing. It just isn't
   realistic.   T   F
7. It's good to weigh yourself every day when you're
   on a diet. That way, you know if you're making
   progress—and you reinforce your success by
   "seeing" it right away.   T   F
8. Strict adherence to a diet is necessary for success.
   If you can't resist a gargantuan dinner on a
   Saturday night and then going out for a hot fudge
   sundae the next night, you might as well forget
   about the whole thing.   T   F

Now, how many of these statements do you consider to be true? My guess is that most people who have been on diets would say that at least five or six of them are true—and probably all of them. In the workshops I conducted, my guess proved correct.

The truth is that all of them are false.

Not only are they false, but if you believe in the truth of even *one* of the statements, that belief in itself could well be responsible for the failure of all your previous dieting efforts.

That is no exaggeration but a very conservatively stated fact, based on innumerable observations by me and by others. If, for instance, you said to yourself, "Yes, my problem is that I need to lose 25 pounds," then I say to you that that one belief has probably undermined and destroyed all your dieting efforts without your ever being aware of why they ultimately failed and why you are overweight today.

If you said to yourself, "True," after reading as few as three or four of the statements, your mental set virtually *guaranteed* that all your previous dieting efforts would fail.

Yet I would guess that these "Deadly Myths," as I call them, are implicit in about nine out of ten dieting books, and that even many doctors would regard most of the statements as true. It's no surprise, then, that losing weight and keeping it off is so difficult.

Embarking on a journey to slenderness with your mind packed with those beliefs is equivalent to setting off on an Arctic exploration believing that the North Pole is a tropical rain forest: You are doomed to failure because you don't understand the territory.

The fundamental reason, then, why the Prevention System of Natural Weight Control is much more likely to succeed than any other reducing plan you have tried is that *we're going to unload these failure-ensuring myths from your mind.*

And as we do that, we are going to replace them, one at a time, with new insights into the reality of weight control. More important, *we're going to arm you with new tools and skills that have been specially designed for successfully coping with weight problems,* just as the gear of an Arctic explorer or a mountain climber is specially designed to cope with his special environment.

To put it another way, the secret of success of this new approach is that there is no diet to follow. Instead of trying to artificially and drastically change the kind and amount of food you're accustomed to eating—an attempt which both of us know is doomed to failure—we are instead going to change *you.*

I don't mean we're going to try to psychoanalyze you or guruize you or change your personality. It's nothing as complicated or as ambitious as that.

What's going to happen as you read this book is that you'll learn some stark truths about weight control that are so obvious—and so important—you'll wonder why so few people seem to be aware of them.

You'll learn how to discover the "hidden" habits that have been defeating all your efforts to control your weight. You'll learn how to change those habits quickly and without using willpower. Intelligence, yes; imagination, yes; perseverance, absolutely—willpower, no.

You'll learn how to get more exercise than you ever dreamed possible—without straining yourself.

You'll learn how to stop being obsessed with food and intimidated by your appetite.

These insights and skills will prove to be more effective than any "diet" yet devised in helping you reach your goals. Soon you'll probably be chuckling to yourself when friend after friend asks you what diet you've been following to lose all that weight.

They just won't believe their ears when you say, "I'm not on a diet."

CHAPTER

2

Dieting and Willpower: Two Things You Don't Need

If you are like most of the people who read and used this book when it was still in the manuscript stage, you probably think it's mighty strange that the statement "My problem is that I need to lose weight" is considered false.

If you get nothing else from this book, you must appreciate the utter falsity—and the hidden trap—in that statement.

And why is it false?

Because, dear reader, if you are like me and 99 out of 100 people who are over 30 and overweight, you have *already* lost weight. It's a safe bet that you have dieted strenuously at least 3 or 4 times and maybe 30 or 40 times. And during at least one of those assaults on your waistline, you probably came very close to reaching your ideal weight. At least, I'd venture, you managed to shed a good 15 pounds or so.

And then what happened?

See what I mean?

If your problem was *truly* that you needed to lose weight, your problem would have been solved a long time ago. It may, in fact, have been solved five times over!

Having lost their weight, at least four out of five dieters immediately revert to the same behavior that got them fat in the first place. And the sad fact is that no matter how many times they go through this cycle, *most dieters never realize that they are guaranteeing their ultimate failure by attacking their bellies instead of their behavior.*

I know. I was there. At 177 pounds, to be exact. And that was a good 25 pounds over where I should have been. Repeated diets worked at first—then failed. Or maybe I should say the diets worked but I failed. Failed to change my behavior. Now I weigh 150, and I've been holding that weight without any great strain for years. What I did was—well, everything you are going to learn in this book.

The idea of changing your behavior may sound difficult or even a little scary. But it isn't. The particular behavior patterns we'll be going after are only those that impinge directly on your weight. For the most part, changing these behavior patterns involves nothing more than modifying certain habits you have—often, habits you don't even know you have. Most people have never even thought twice about these habits—perhaps not even once, because a number of them are performed almost unconsciously.

But how does one go about changing habits, anyway? Especially when you may not even be aware that you have them? The answer is through the use of those *tools* and *skills* we mentioned before.

Most of us would regard our bodies as being at least as important as our houses. Yet, when it comes to remodeling the body, we usually go about the project as if it were some silly game instead of a major project the success of which could bring us enormous gratification and heightened enjoyment of living.

We attack the job with no skills or tools whatsoever. And the only blueprint we have—in most cases—is a greased-lightning miracle diet published in a magazine or maybe one from that endless series of diet books.

Oh, we *do* have one tool that we count on in our endless dieting, and we use it until it snaps under the strain—*willpower.*

Using willpower as your chief tool in dieting is like trying to drive nails into wood with your bare fists.

Combined with other qualities and assets—most of them new habits—willpower may have a place in the scheme of things after all.

But to rely on it exclusively is probably the greatest mistake that any weight-reducer could ever make.

Now that we've come to grips with yet another of the "Deadly Myths" of dieting, let me add that the concept of willpower *in general* is highly overrated. I know that no one ever wrote a poem or built a sailboat or closed a big sale or raised three children on the strength of willpower. What is willpower, anyway, but an unceasing spasm of negativity? Desire, perseverance, patience and the right skills are the kinds of assets that get important things done. That goes for losing weight, too.

WHY CRASH DIETING
MAKES US FATTER IN THE END

Any temporary, quick-fix weight-loss scheme is doomed to fail. And it will probably make you fat, too. That's what Kelly Brownell, Ph.D., who researches obesity at the University of Pennsylvania in Philadelphia, found when he investigated the effects of such yo-yo dieting. "Some patients have trouble losing weight despite low calorie intakes, sometimes as low as 700 or 800 calories a day," says Dr. Brownell. "We noticed that this problem was more common in people who had been on many diets in the past. So we wondered if calorie restriction could actually make dieting more difficult by reducing calorie needs."

To find out, he made a bunch of rats into yo-yo dieters. He fed them high-fat diets until they were pudgy, then put them on two cycles of dieting down to normal size and then regaining all that weight.

And it turned out that dieting *did* make their bodies hold on to fat stubbornly. "During their first diet, the yo-yo rats took 21 days to get down to normal weight," says Dr. Brownell. "The second diet took 46 days for the same weight loss, on exactly the same caloric intake!"

And the rats gained weight even more quickly. After their first diet, it took 45 days to get fat again. The second regaining period was only 14 days.

(continued)

WHY CRASH DIETING MAKES
US FATTER IN THE END—*Continued*

Bad news for fat rats. But do humans have the same plight? It looks like the answer is yes. Two recent studies at Harvard University showed that people who went on a very low-calorie diet, gained weight and then went on the diet again lost less weight the second time around.

It might seem that your body is trying to thwart you. But actually, it thinks it's saving your life. It thinks you're starving. So to protect you from the repeated famines, it gets really good at storing up fat. It slows down your metabolism and tries to put every calorie to use.

THE RIGHT WAY TO LOSE WEIGHT

Meanwhile, even if you've been a diet junky, don't give up hope. No matter how many diets you've endured, you can still lose weight. It might take a long time, but it's possible.

"My studies may sound gloomy, but they do imply two positive recommendations," says Dr. Brownell. "For one, you have to take dieting seriously. Don't just try to lose weight on a New Year's resolution or a whim, because you'll probably regain the weight. Wait until you're fully committed.

"Second, find a good program that focuses on gradual, permanent change and that attempts to maintain your new behaviors. You should eat a low-fat, high-fiber diet moderately low in calories. And exercise regularly."

The choice is yours. Develop healthy, reasonable eating habits and keep weight off permanently—or become a frustrated yo-yo.

3

Reshape
Your Eating Style

Did you ever wonder *why* you eat too much?

Most people of whom I ask this question reply with an answer something like one of these:

"My appetite is too big."

"I'm a glutton, I suppose."

"I guess I'm just hungry all the time!"

Would your answer be similar? Do you think that your hunger is some kind of mad, starving beast? Well, relax; it isn't.

What if I told you that a very substantial amount of your eating is done without any sense of hunger whatsoever?

What effect would it have on your attitude toward your eating problem to know that it is perfectly possible for you to eat substantially less than you do now and never once get into a brawl with a hungry stomach? Would it make you feel *good?*

All of us are familiar with some instances where we eat even though we're not particularly hungry. Sometimes we may be absolutely stuffed, but we still go on eating. Usually, we think of this happening when we are enjoying a very special meal at a fine restaurant in the company of good friends, or perhaps a Thanksgiving dinner. That kind of once-in-a-while indulgence is nothing to worry about. But few of us seem to realize that *eating when we're not really hungry is something we do almost every single day of our lives.* Eating without hunger is so commonplace that we do it almost unconsciously, and for a very wide range of reasons.

If you want to lose weight and keep it off, it is absolutely essential for you to become aware of when, where and why you are eating without hunger. *Once you have identified this behavior, you have at the same time found a wonderful opportunity for reducing your intake of food without fighting your hunger or depriving yourself of needed nourishment.* In the next chapter, I'll begin to arm you with the skills you need to change your behavior and take advantage of this opportunity, but before I do that, you must become aware of exactly what it is you are going to change.

SPOTTING PATTERNS
OF EATING BEHAVIOR

One of the first things I did in a series of diet workshops that I ran some time ago was to ask all the participants to keep a daily log of what they ate. But the important thing was not the total amount of what they ate—since everyone's caloric needs are different—but when, where and under what circumstances they ate.

We also asked each participant to write down exactly how he felt before, during and after each instance of eating, whether it was a meal, a major snack or simply a quick nibble of this or that.

Each reader would be well advised to do the same thing for himself, but experience tells me that precious few people are actually going to do that. So instead, we'll review the experiences of our workshop participants in the expectation that each reader will probably be able to spot his own behavior patterns reflected in those of the participants.

Way out in front as the occasion for eating without hunger was snacking while watching TV, generally between the hours of 8:30 and 11:00 P.M.

"As soon as the first or second commercial goes on for the movie of the night, I get an uncontrollable desire to raid the refrigerator," one woman said, and at least half the other participants nodded their heads vigorously.

"Do you feel hunger at that time?"

"No, not at all. It's only been about 2 hours since I've finished eating dinner." Again, many of the other participants nodded.

"In between programs," another woman said, "I get an uncontrollable urge to get a bowl of pretzels and potato chips, set them down in front of me, and munch away."

"Do you feel hunger at that time?"

"To tell you the truth, sometimes I can still feel my dinner digesting in my stomach, but that doesn't seem to matter."

In fact, all the participants admitted that before TV snacking, they definitely were not hungry in the sense that their stomachs were uncomfortable, let alone growling.

In my own case, when I examined when and why I was eating, I realized that the desire for food was not coming from my stomach at all, but from my head. Even more specifically, it often seemed to stem from my *mouth*. Somewhere between the hours of about 8:00 P.M. and midnight, I would—sometimes more than once—get a kind of dissatisfaction or itchiness or uneasiness and—entirely without thinking about what was going on—I would habitually start flinging open pantry doors, gazing inside the refrigerator and taking quick looks inside the freezer.

Further reflection revealed that after eating whatever I chose (which meant whatever was handy), I rarely felt satisfied in any meaningful way. Rather, I felt uncomfortable. Ironically, even though I would often be uncomfortable, I would also feel a desire to eat still *more* food. Why, I'm not exactly sure, except that my digestive processes apparently swung into action after tasting the snack and protested being trifled with.

Many workshop participants said they typically nibbled on food while they were preparing dinner. It wasn't that they were really hungry or that they couldn't wait to sit down for the meal, but just having their fingers in all that food made it seem somehow logical to slip a few mouthfuls of this and that down the hatch.

In fact, whether or not it occurred while cooking, a surprising amount of eating without hunger proved to be taking place either at the kitchen counter or right in front of an open refrigerator. Clearly, the mere proximity of food is motive enough to put it into your mouth, just as if the tonsils were a powerful magnet and the food, iron filings. Honest-to-goodness hunger often has nothing to do with it.

Several participants said that they ate when they were not hungry because their spouses were eating (whether *they* were actually hungry or not is another story), and they felt that it was unfriendly or uncooperative to refuse to share a snack. The temptation to do this is especially strong among people who may not spend a great deal of time with their spouses. Since all our workshop participants—the overwhelming number of whom were women—worked every day, these little moments of sharing probably had a special value. Still, the bottom line is that *they were eating when they were not hungry.*

DEALING WITH THE HABIT FACTOR

One of the most common causes of eating without hunger—real, physical hunger—is loneliness or depression. There is something about the act of eating that is a kind of balm for these negative feelings, albeit a very transitory balm. What's more, a person conditioned by habit to eat without hunger almost never chooses healthful food at these moments. Almost invariably, it is cake, pie, ice cream or chocolate— something *sweet*. Which means, of course, something very high in calories.

Eating triggered by loneliness can be a powerful reflex, but although *everyone* feels lonely or depressed from time to time, not everyone eats in response to these negative emotions. It follows that reflexive eating without hunger in response to these emotions is a *learned* behavior, not an instinctive behavior, and can therefore be *unlearned*. Even better, because eating does nothing in the long run to solve loneliness or depression, that kind of behavior can be replaced by more positive actions that enhance your ego as they diminish your hips.

Many workshop participants reported that after keeping a diary for a few days, they realized a major cause of eating without hunger was simple boredom. Eating, besides everything else you can say about it, is, after all, something to do. And food processors use every trick in the book to give food amusement value. They make snacks very crunchy and very salty, and then imbue them with exotic artifi- cial flavors and colors. Soda pop and other beverages have a high amusement value. Popcorn, while certainly not a junk food, can nevertheless be abused when it is eaten not as a snack when you are hungry but simply because you are bored and feel that your teeth and tongue need something to play with.

Ritualistic overeating on special occasions seems to be natural and is nothing to worry about, really. But many of us have a way of promoting every possible event to "special occasion" status. At one company where I worked, it was traditional for members of the office staff to bring in cakes on the occasion of someone's birthday. Somehow, these treats were always super-rich productions like Dutch chocolate cake. If there was no cake, there was bound to be something like custard-filled doughnuts. That meant that about a dozen times a year, most of the office staff was indulging in 300 or 400 calories—even though they weren't the least bit hungry, as these cakes were generally served at about 10:00 A.M. Eventually the custom stopped, apparently for two reasons. First, many people became concerned about this pointless eating without hunger, and second, a number of office workers were getting headaches or attacks of reactive low blood sugar in the wake of eating rich cakes and pastries in the morning.

Another version of the same general phenomenon often occurs when people visit each other's homes, not for major occasions but simply for a brief social visit. At these times, it is often considered mandatory for the host or hostess to serve up vast quantities of food, nearly always including pastries and cakes. More likely than not, the people indulging in this food are not really hungry and would be content with a cup of coffee, but the combination of social ritual and the sheer physical presence of heaps of food piled in front of them triggers yet another instance of eating without hunger.

In the next few chapters, I'm going to teach you how to avoid eating without hunger. At least I'm going to try. But before I do that, I'd like you to answer the following questions.

1. Did any of the instances of eating without hunger sound familiar to you?
2. Did any of those instances seem *very* familiar?
3. If you had a minute to think about it, could you come up with at least one personal example of eating without hunger I *didn't* mention? (Like eating the kids' leftovers . . . eating

the potato chips that unexpectedly came with the hamburger you ordered . . . eating popcorn at the movies?)
4. Does it seem to you that eating is too important to your health and well-being to be carried out in a semiconscious state?

If you answered yes to all of the above questions, you are now ready to learn how to change your behavior.

CHAPTER

4

If You Really Want It, Eat It!

Remember the old saw about counting to ten before saying anything in anger?

The idea behind that musty adage is that most impulses to swear or yell at someone are so fleeting that if you simply think about something else for a little while, they will evaporate. And why bring down the wrath of the Almighty or lose a friend because of a fleeting impulse?

Nowadays, swearing isn't considered terribly sinful, while speaking out sharply is often said to be downright therapeutic. But when it comes to *eating* on impulse, no change in social customs can excuse the calories consumed.

And what this short but important chapter is going to do is simply teach you a fancy way of counting to ten before you give in to a fleeting impulse to push something into your mouth.

Let's say you're cruising by the refrigerator and, lo and behold, the door flings itself open. My, isn't that cup of custard interesting?

Very interesting. And you know what? I'm hungry! I mean, really. After all, didn't I skip breakfast . . . the day before yesterday? . . . Ooo, but I'm supposed to be losing weight . . . .But I'm hungry, dammit! I can eat when I'm *hungry,* can't I?

When you get into a situation like that, you're in trouble. Because one thing most people can't stand is to feel *deprived.* And no matter how fleeting the eating impulse may be, it usually gets its way by mounting a horse called "I really deserve this!" Here's what to do when you are confronted with that classic situation:

Tell yourself that if you are *really* hungry, you can certainly eat. All you have to do is wait 7 minutes. Close the refrigerator door, knowing that the food is still going to be there 7 minutes later, and then go do something else. Open a magazine, listen to some music, do anything you want to, as long as it gets you out of the kitchen or whatever room the confrontation occurs in.

Seven minutes later, if you still want that food, go and eat it. Maybe you really *are* hungry. Maybe not, but eating at that point may well be better for your reducing program than feeling deprived.

That delaying tactic, or balk, as baseball fans might like to call it, is one of the standard techniques taught by many behavioral psychologists treating people with eating problems. Different practitioners recommend different waiting times, but I have chosen 7 minutes because if the delay is a round figure like 10 minutes, there is a tendency to regard it as a concept rather than 10 actual minutes: "I'll just wait a little while and then go eat it." If you think like that, "a little while" is liable to turn out to be 30 seconds. In practice, I've found that 7 minutes is usually time enough to do the job, yet not so long as to be intimidating.

But even more important than really waiting 7 minutes is to understand that the idea of this delay is not to somehow "trick" you out of your desired food. All you're doing is *testing* your impulse to see if it's sincere. If it is, act on it with an easy conscience. You haven't lost at any game. Whether you eat it or not, you've won, because you've done it *your way.*

One woman said this technique was the same idea parents try to get across to their teenage daughters when they are the recipients of sweaty propositions. "It's a question of self-respect," the workshop participant said. I like that.

WINNING WITHOUT WILLPOWER

Let's now take a slow-motion look at the "showdown" at the refrigerator, to better understand what's really happening, and come up with some special moves we can utilize in executing the 7-minute delay technique.

There you were, walking through the kitchen, and the next thing you knew, you had opened the refrigerator door. Were you *hungry* when you opened the refrigerator? Hungry, shmungry, just about every time you pass that refrigerator you open it, don't you? And *why?* The answer is easy: it's a *habit!*

Right now I want you to get an image of yourself opening the refrigerator door and looking inside. As you see yourself in your mind's eye, realize that what you are doing is an unconscious—or at best, semiconscious—habit. You are acting like a laboratory mouse that spends half its waking hours making meaningless gestures like pressing a lever because it has been conditioned to do so. Now see an image of yourself as a giant laboratory mouse standing on its hind legs looking into your refrigerator, twitching its nose like crazy and reaching out for food because a graduate student in psychology has taught it to do so whether it is hungry or not. *How do you like being a mouse?*

Actually, it's no great disgrace to do something out of habit. We do it all the time, when we nod at people, smile, straighten a stack of papers or begin singing as soon as we step into the shower.

The difference between doing those things and opening the refrigerator door and snatching food is that smiling at people and singing in the shower aren't harmful. In fact, they're probably *good* habits. Most important, singing in the shower never increased the size of anyone's rear end the way grabbing food from the refrigerator does.

Picture yourself as a giant mouse again, nose quivering, eyes all beady, standing in front of the refrigerator. Picture it vividly . . . then let it slowly dissolve from your consciousness.

Suddenly it's *you* standing in front of the refrigerator. Intelligent, hard-working you. The apex of evolution. Made in God's image. Any way you look at it, that's a mighty big brain you've got tucked inside your skull. A creature quite like you came up with the theory of relativity, discovered the atom, wrote *Don Quixote* and figured out how to eradicate smallpox from the face of the earth. There you are, in all your majestic humanity, standing in front of the refrigerator eyeballing a cup of custard.

Somewhere in your brain is the knowledge that losing the blubber on your body is one of the most important things you can do to enjoy a happier future. The day your weight begins to go down, in fact, every moment of your life will be happier. Every day you will become healthier. Every day you will increase your energy and endurance. Every day you will become more attractive to yourself and to your friends. But the part of the brain that knows this is not the only part of your nervous system that's working. In fact, the habit part, the semiconscious part, is red-hot. The mouse part of you. The part that does things without thinking, the part that keeps you eating when you don't want to eat.

It's very undignified, really. Who wants to fight a mouse? So do what any self-respecting Homo sapiens would do: Simply walk away, instantly causing that mouse to disappear. It's not a willpower struggle, really, because as you leave the scene, you make a mental note that you will renegotiate the entire matter in precisely 7 minutes. (Unless, of course, you are then otherwise engaged. I mean, why go out of your way to keep an appointment with a mouse?)

Clop. The refrigerator door just closed.

Klack. The door of the kitchen cabinet is shut.

Clong. That was the top of the cookie jar.

Now what? Without any further ado, not even a little dab of ado, haul your bones out of the kitchen.

TAKING TIME OUT

What you do next depends on your individual interests. Do you love music? Get out your favorite record, slip it on the turntable and listen to a couple of songs. But do it with a little finesse. If your favorite tune is the fourth cut on side A, put the needle at the beginning of the record. Now if after 7 minutes you want to take the record off before it gets to the part you like most, fine. That's part of the bargain. Like I said, you won't be losing, or suffering any kind of defeat. But maybe, just maybe, you'll find yourself wanting to hear your favorite part of the record a little more than you want that custard. In fact, there's a possibility that after 5 minutes or so, you'll have forgotten about that custard completely. You may not even think about it again until you go to bed, when the whole incident will bring a very self-satisfied smirk to your face.

Like to read? Find a new magazine or book, take it into the living room or bedroom and plunge right in. Have you noticed that lately you haven't been able to find time to do the reading you really want to do? Well, you've just found that time.

Or maybe there's something in the workshop or in the sewing basket that you've been wanting to do for a couple of weeks. Here's the chance you've been waiting for. A very special kind of time that is reserved for doing exactly and exclusively what you want to do most. Oil your gun. Hang a picture. Paint a picture. Sit on your husband's lap. Teach your dog a new trick. Carry out the trash. Do the laundry. The ironing. Call your sister. See how many sit-ups you can do. Take the dog for a walk. Write a letter to your son. A letter to the editor. Vacuum the rugs. Get out the Sears catalog and decide what clothing you're going to buy when you lose your first 10 pounds.

My brother Barry, a psychotherapist, advises people who want to lose weight to find a new hobby and really get involved in it. You can see why. If you have nothing to turn to except your TV, you're going to be in trouble. Because TV doesn't involve you the way real activities do. The first time a commercial break flashes on the screen, you're apt to say "Time's up!" and run back to the refrigerator or the cookie jar.

The activity you choose may be something you've been pursuing casually for quite a while. In the back of your mind, you've had the idea that it would really be fun to go at this hobby flat out, and if that's the case, now's the time to stomp on the accelerator. Buy the latest books about it. Go shopping for new equipment. Join a club. Tackle a really challenging but satisfying project.

You see, having a hobby is worth a lot more to you as a person with an eating problem than merely filling in 7 minutes' time. In my own case, the hobby or interest that I took up when I went on a weight-reducing program was jogging. Now, of course, any kind of exercise hobby is going to be doubly valuable, because it burns up calories while it keeps your mind busy. When I got into jogging, I got into it *mentally* as well as physically. When I wasn't running, I was often thinking about it. I would read *Runner's World,* not just once but two or three times. I even daydreamed about running. In short, as my brother Barry put it, I was "obsessed" with it. And he thought this was important because people who are trying to reduce often become obsessed with *food*—if they weren't before. And if you walk around all day thinking about food, you're going to be excruciatingly vulnerable to its charms, real or imagined. You're much better off daydreaming about swimming or quilting or building the addition on your home or having your sheepdog win Best in Show.

One of the best obsessions to become a prisoner of is gardening. I would recommend it emphatically for anyone who has an eating problem during the day. Gardening not only gets you out of the kitchen, it gets you out of the house. It gives you exercise, and perhaps most important of all, it gets your hands dirty. Hobbies that keep your hands busy, dirty, greasy or wet, and therefore unable to reach into the refrigerator, are the best hobbies of all. During the evening, you can lavish loving attention on your pet, your indoor plants, your sculpturing or oil painting.

The best part about this whole approach is that you've used a no-win confrontation between food and willpower as a springboard to launch you into activities that will not only help you lose weight but will add a lot of enjoyment to your life and make you feel much better about yourself.

5

How to Make Weight Loss Easier

No matter what kind of work we hope to do, we can make it easier on ourselves if we get organized first.

If it's tools we're going to need, we get them together and put them within easy reach. If the work we are going to do involves moving from place to place, we remove everything blocking efficient movement—first. Imagine, for a moment, what it would be like to try to do a household job with your tools scattered all over the house, the garage and the yard. Or imagine trying to play tennis with beer cans and newspapers scattered all over the court.

If *those* examples seem silly, imagine how silly it is to try to do something as important as losing a substantial amount of weight without first getting yourself organized. Yet that is exactly what most of us (including me) have done in the past, with the predictable result of stumbling over all sorts of impediments . . . and finally getting so angry and frustrated that we simply give up.

Think of your weight-loss program as a journey. There is a long road ahead of you. But fortunately, right now, you can decide whether that is going to be a road full of potholes, bumps, debris and unmarked turns, or a well-paved, well-lit, well-marked path to success.

Sure, if you try hard enough, you can get there just the same, but which would you rather be, an engineer or a human bulldozer?

STRATEGIES THAT WORK

You already have at your disposal a lot of the information you'll need to engineer a smoother path to weight loss and permanent weight control. That information consists of a knowledge of your own eating habits. You've become aware of the fact that a lot of the eating you do is carried out in what I call a semiconscious state and is not motivated by real hunger but simply by habit and shallow impulses. Then you learned how to change some of those habits and how to *test* those impulses to find out if they are legitimate or phony. What we are going to do in this chapter is learn how to make it *easier* to change those habits and reduce the number of phony impulses we have to contend with.

Localize your eating.   You have already thought about circumstances that lead you to eat, other than mealtime. Now I want you to think about *where* you eat, other than your dining room table. We asked the participants in our workshop to do this, and here are some of their answers.

"I do 90 percent of my snacking sitting on the sofa watching the TV," Marie said. Many others nodded in agreement.

"Standing right in front of the refrigerator," Stan said. "It is amazing how much I can eat, just standing there. Sometimes I don't even close the door. I keep the door open with the elbow of the same arm I'm using to eat!"

"At the kitchen counter, usually when I'm preparing dinner."

"I like to eat in bed, and there is nothing I like better than to eat crackers with peanut butter while I'm reading."

"This may sound strange, but I like to eat most when I'm driving. I'll stop into a Seven-Eleven store and buy some cupcakes or maybe a whole box of cookies and eat them while I'm driving."

Some people eat more than they need to, and frequently more than they want to, when they're eating dinner. We will get to that challenge a little later, but by far the greatest amount of impulse eating occurs *between* meals and is almost always done at places *other* than the table where meals are eaten.

You've already made a deal with yourself that if you are *really* hungry, you can have the food. So what we are going to do now is give you a new way to further "legitimize" your eating. Make this new deal with yourself: If you have decided that you really want to eat something, and if you have waited 7 minutes after your initial eating impulse, you may eat it *only* if you do so seated at your dining room table.

There is no deprivation of food involved here. Far from it. Instead, you are going to enjoy your food in proper fashion. Whatever it is you have decided to eat, put it on a plate or in a bowl, take it to the dining room table, sit down and thoroughly enjoy every mouthful. I guarantee that doing this will not increase the caloric content of your snack one bit; gobbling your food in front of the refrigerator is every bit as fattening as eating it from Bavarian china set on Spanish linen on your French provincial table.

Why go to all that trouble? Precisely because it is trouble. Going through that routine forces you to become acutely conscious of what you are doing. If your desire for food is legitimate and not merely part of some mindless habit pattern like eating crackers while you watch TV in bed, it will not seem like any great ordeal to set the table and eat as if you really mean it. But if you are only kidding yourself, it may well seem like more trouble than it is worth. And often, that is exactly what happens.

Remember, the idea behind this is not to deprive you of food that you really want, but only to make sure that you really want it. Surely, if you really want it, spending a single minute serving your food in a normal way is not unreasonable. And when you eat, you may do so with an absolutely easy conscience, because in all likelihood, your desire for that food is legitimate: hunger, not habit.

When you eat . . . eat! Now that you have become more conscious about *where* you eat, consider this question: Do you ever engage in snacking or even full-scale eating while you are doing something else? Or, looking at it another way, do you do anything *else* while you are eating? If so, what?

"I play cards once a week, and I just love to snack while I play," Sally said.

"With me, it's watching TV, just like before," Marie said. "TV is more enjoyable when you are eating."

"Sometimes the programs are so dumb!" Roberta added.

"I always eat popcorn when I go to the movies."

"I always have a couple of beers when I go bowling."

"I know it is bad manners, but I almost always read the newspaper while I'm eating dinner."

Do any of those responses sound familiar? Maybe you have your own special activities that seem to invite snacking. With me, as with some of the others, it was watching TV. Whether it was just a simple habit or, like Roberta said, because the programs are usually so dumb, I can't say. Perhaps it was simply a habit left over from my childhood, when I used to eat dinner from a TV tray while watching cartoons or football games. In any event, there is no doubt that many of us employ eating as a kind of background music while we are doing something else, much as the smoker lights up when he gets into a heavy conversation or goes to a cocktail party.

So let's make another deal. If you are doing something other than sitting down to a meal, and you want to eat, you certainly can—but only if you stop what you're doing, go to the dining room table as before, and sit down and eat *while doing nothing other than eating.* If you're *really* hungry, you'll do it. If not, you won't. You'll prefer to keep on playing cards or watching the football game or reading your book.

As a kind of corollary to this principle, I must advise strongly against reading at the table. The more conscious you are of eating, the better off you will be. Your food will be much more satisfying when you are paying attention to it, looking at it, smelling it, feeling it, tasting it, chewing it, thinking about it.

When do you lose control? This next little bit of domestic engineering is related to those above but asks the specific question, At what point in your daily schedule, or what time of the day, do you seem to do the most snacking? More than likely, it's the evening. Perhaps it occurs when you are watching TV, as mentioned before, but right now I want you to think about the problem in a slightly broader perspective. In other words, it might be more effective to look upon a certain part of the day as your vulnerable *time,* rather than a vulnerable activity or place. Now, if you are in fact doing most of your snacking in the evening, say between the hours of 9:00 P.M. and 11:00 P.M., why not plan on *scheduling* some new kind of activity during those hours, something to reduce the total number of phony eating impulses you have to contend with? You could, for instance, schedule several evening trips to the Y every week, sign up for classes or clubs that meet at night, take up a new hobby or rekindle your interest in an old one that can take you away from all the familiar cues, like watching TV, that habitually spark those snacking impulses.

With me, the vulnerable time was between the hours of 11:00 P.M. and 1:00 A.M. Usually, at that time, I'd be through my evening reading and writing and would watch TV until I couldn't keep my eyes open anymore. It was amazing how many trips I used to make to the refrigerator. There was no legitimate reason for me to be that hungry, so I thought about exactly what it was that was causing me to do all that uncontrollable snacking.

The major reason, I concluded, was simply that when it's late at night and I'm tired, the most rational part of my mind rapidly becomes drugged. I'm a sucker for any fleeting impulse. But there might have been another reason, I concluded, and that was that I was eating in a kind of perverted attempt to stay awake. By shoveling sweet things down my throat, I caused my blood sugar to rise and give me a temporary energy boost. Then I asked myself, *Why am I staying up so late in the first place?* Why is it so important to watch those old movies I have seen so many times, or see who the next celebrity is going to be on the Johnny Carson show, when all it's doing for me is making me incredibly tired and causing me to eat like a maniac? I didn't have any answer to that.

Finally I got the idea of simply cutting those late hours out of my life, like hacking off a rotten limb from a tree, and replacing them with a couple of other hours during which I would be fresh, totally in control of my impulses and not in the least inclined to snack. In other words, I started going to bed at 11:00 P.M. and waking up at 6:30, instead of going to bed at 1:00 A.M. and waking up at 8:00.

And that was one of the smartest things I ever did.

I was able to avoid a lot of impulse eating without getting into a "confrontation" with the food, I felt much more rested in the morning, and I found the new time I had created for myself in the morning to be ideal for jogging or writing, which I did on alternate days.

Out of sight, maybe out of mind.   Have you ever found yourself eating something simply because it was *there?* I mean *right* there— smack under your nose. I guess we all have. Many of us impulse eaters are something like frogs, programmed by evolution to flick out their tongues whenever anything small enough to be slurped down moves into range of vision.

Why make it difficult on yourself by permitting all sorts of unwanted foods to entice you? If you really *want* food, you know where to get it. The idea is to keep it from *harassing* you.

What I suggest, therefore, is that you spend 10 minutes or so doing a little redecorating and moving. Are there bowls of chips or pretzels or candies scattered around your house? Maybe they *do* add an interesting note of warmth or color to the decor, but imagine what they're going to do for the decor of your belly and hips. Get rid of them. Wrap them up and put them away. That even goes for bowls of fruit. Fruit is a good food, but no food, no matter how nourishing, should be eaten on the merest of impulses, simply because it is *there*.

What about your kitchen counter? Are there boxes of crackers or cookies? Packages of doughnuts? English muffins? Sweetened cereal? Perhaps a bottle of wine? Take a good, hard look.

I want you to put all those things away, but not just anyplace. Take all of them and put them in one special cabinet or drawer, which will be, in effect, a fat-food compound. Preferably, this should be a cabinet that's a little bit out of your way or hard to reach. You won't be opening it by accident. And by having all those snacks in one place, instead of merely hiding them in the back of your regular cabinets, you won't be "accidentally" stumbling across a bag of pretzels while you're hunting for a can of tomato sauce.

But what about the kids? some people ask. They have to be able to get these snacks easily, don't they? To which I answer, *Why?* Do they really *need* potato chips, pretzels, candy and all those other empty-calorie foods? Maybe *they* think they do, but you know better. I'm not saying they can *never* have any pretzels or chips, only that they, too, should be conscious of what they are putting into their mouths. And it seems to me that if your children are so small that they can't reach food placed in a cabinet, then they ought to be *asking* you if they may have a snack in the first place.

As for the refrigerator, it would be nice if we could all afford two refrigerators, but lacking that, we can at least keep things arranged so that the high-calorie impulse items are consistently placed way in the back. Let's face it, even if you are abiding by your agreement not to grab anything out of the refrigerator until you've waited 7 minutes, you're going to be making it that much easier on yourself if, when you *do* have to open the refrigerator for a legitimate reason, the first thing you see isn't a half-eaten blueberry pie ringed by bottles of Coca-Cola.

The front of your refrigerator should be loaded with fruits, vegetables and meat-and-potato-type leftovers. Likewise, the storage shelves on the inside of your refrigerator door should be restricted to carrying nonsnack items like eggs and butter. In the freezer compartment, put any ice cream or similar snacks behind the frozen meats and vegetables.

Signs of the new times. Now that you have done some engineering to make the road to permanent slenderness a little smoother, give some attention to helpful road signs. These road signs—you may be using anywhere from one to half a dozen—will be placed throughout your home, in places where there are critical "turns." I know it sounds a little corny, but many people find that domestic signs prove every bit as useful in preventing needless wrong turns as the road signs on a busy freeway. In fact, that's a good analogy, because just as a highway sign sort of jogs you out of the semihypnotic state that you sometimes fall into when zooming down the road mile after mile, a domestic sign can suddenly restore you to full consciousness as you drive down the road of daily routine.

7 MINUTES. THANK YOU!

That was the sign one workshop participant placed on her refrigerator door. She reported it cut down the number of times she opened the door by about 25 percent. A man put a sign on his refrigerator door that read:

ARE YOU HONESTLY HUNGRY? FIND OUT

The sign I put in my own kitchen, taped to a cabinet and written in large, colorful letters, was:

EAT IT AT THE TABLE, PLEASE

Notice that I'm not suggesting you put up signs saying things like "Don't eat it!" or "Do you want to stay fat?" For one thing, I don't believe much in negativity, or in threats, either. It's hard enough putting up with the negativity and harassment of others, so why should we have to insult *ourselves?* Be intelligent, polite; show respect for yourself.

I suggested to one woman who was having a difficult time getting into the habit of walking that, among other things, she put a sign on her coat-closet door reading:

WANT TO LOSE SOME WEIGHT, RIGHT NOW?

But the sign she actually *did* put up read:

WEIGHT-LOSS EQUIPMENT ROOM

Use your imagination to decide what kind of signs you're going to use. In fact, spending a few moments at this will give you the added benefit of raising your consciousness of those places in your home where you're especially vulnerable. If you feel, for example, that you might "accidentally" fling open the cabinet door where you've stashed away snacks, label it with a sign reading simply:

FAT-FOOD COMPOUND

Or:

DRINK SOME WATER!

Or maybe just:

THINK!

One sign that sounds a little simplistic but really isn't, is:

THINK THIN!

What that sign means is just what it says. Think that you *are* thin. Picture yourself as a slender person, an active person, a person with a perfectly normal appetite. It's a little bit like the hypnotic technique of imagining, for instance, that the pain *is* gone, which seems to be more effective than imagining that it's beginning to go away. Along these lines, I like the signs that Linda put up, the first on the inside of her front door, the second in her bedroom:

HOME OF THE WORLD'S CHAMPION WALKER
EVERY DAY I AM A NEW PERSON

Help your family help you. An absolutely incredible amount of eating without hunger is done for the simple reason that someone else in the family offers you food. I don't mean when they serve you a meal, but when they invite you to eat more than *you've* decided to eat, or at a time when you aren't particularly interested in eating. At the table, many of us say to our spouses or children things like:

"Want some more spaghetti?"

"Don't you like my muffins? They're delicious!"

"Finish your potatoes, Billy."

"Want to split that last piece of pie with me?"

"Is that all you're going to eat?"

If people are really hungry, if they really need more food, they don't have to be cajoled or even invited to eat it. When you invite them to do more eating, you are interfering with the functioning of their natural appetite control system, which is the most fundamental mistake that can be made.

But what if other people keep pushing food at *you*? Probably that's happening, and maybe more than you think. Wives do it, husbands do it, neighbors do it, hosts do it, and sometimes waiters do it. The only people who *don't* do it are children, who have more common sense than we give them credit for. But if it's inappropriate for a child to encourage an adult to eat more, it's just as inappropriate—and perhaps even more inexcusable—for one adult to push food at another.

Therefore, what I suggest is that you simply ask other members of your household not to offer you food. Explain to them that you've decided to slim down and that the program you're following depends on not eating when you're not hungry. So to help you, would they please refrain from offering you second helpings, snacks, glasses of wine, even pieces of fruit.

At first, they will probably slip up. When they do, don't get angry. Just say, "No thanks, I don't want to eat when I'm not really hungry." That will gently remind them of what you told them before, without explicitly criticizing them. And you don't want to criticize anyone in your household at this time, because that will only increase the tension and make your new way of eating more difficult. The idea is to make it easy on yourself!

CHAPTER

6

Water Your Body and Grow Thin

By now, we all know that many of our impulses to eat are not triggered by true hunger but by nonphysical factors ranging from a desire to be polite to a need to keep our hands busy. I'm sure many people realize that without having read this book.

But what most people do not realize is that a major reason for irrational eating behavior is the failure to recognize that *many impulses to eat something are misinterpretations of thirst—a desire, a real honest-to-goodness need, for water.*

Your body's need for H_2O is more urgent than its need for any other compound except O_2—oxygen. Two or three days without water is enough to put anyone at death's door, while a single day without water can endanger the life of someone who is not in robust health. Intestinal infections causing diarrhea take the lives of more infants throughout the world than any other disease; death is caused not by the bacteria per se but by dehydration. It is entirely logical, then, that *nature has endowed us with an extraordinarily powerful thirst mechanism to ensure that we get enough of this vital fluid.*

The big problem as far as our health and our waistlines are concerned is that *what we do when this thirst mechanism goes into operation is not what nature intended us to do.*

I became aware of that shortly after I began the weight-control program described in this book. When I had an impulse to put something into my mouth when it wasn't time for a meal, I would wait for 7 minutes or so and then observe what happened to the put-something-in-my-mouth impulse over that short stretch of time. But I did something else, too. Instead of just closing the refrigerator door and going down to my basement to listen to music, I would stand there for a while and try to analyze the exact nature of the impulse that had caused me to open the refrigerator door almost unconsciously.

When you're trying to analyze that kind of impulse, you may not have much success if you're too aggressive or direct in your analysis. So I did what I often do when confronted by a problem at work or in my personal life: I simply emptied my mind, slipping into a kind of instant meditation, but remaining sensitive to images, thoughts or feelings that seemed to thrust themselves into my consciousness.

And when I did that, it dawned on me that the basic need that had taken me to the refrigerator was *dryness of my mouth and throat.*

What an amazing revelation that was! There I was, in the so-familiar posture: poised before the refrigerator door, my eyes wandering over the lighted contents, trying to decide what I felt like eating. What I *really* wanted—the desire that had brought me there—was not anything at all to be found in the refrigerator, but simply *water.*

But then—*why had I gone to the refrigerator?*

That was no great mystery, at least on one level of understanding. It was conditioned response to a sensation of oral uneasiness that I had never before bothered to reflect upon. In other words, a stupid habit.

There's another reason, though, why we are able to habitually eat when our bodies want us to drink, and still not run into problems with dehydration. And that is that *many foods, including most of our favorite snacks, consist largely of water.*

A piece of apple pie, for instance, is by weight almost 48 percent water.

Cheddar cheese is 37 percent water.

Boston creme pie is 35 percent water.

Chocolate cake is 25 percent water.

Chocolate pudding is 65 percent water.

Potato salad, for all its calories, is 76 percent water.

Fruits such as cherries, apples and peaches are between 80 and 90 percent water.

Even chicken and beef contain a lot of water—averaging about 60 percent.

Ice cream is 63 percent water.

After running the above information through my head, I decided that the next time I found myself clutching the refrigerator door, I was going to shuffle over a few steps, turn on the faucet and draw myself a big glass of cold water. Eureka! It was incredibly satisfying—even more so than sweet snacks, because water was what my body wanted and now I was giving it *the real thing!*

Each of you must figure out for yourself how you are going to get good water and how you are going to get into the habit of drinking it. For many, this will prove to be remarkably easy. For others, it may mean buying a water filter or bottled spring water in order to get something that you can really enjoy drinking. It may also mean keeping a supply of clean, attractive drinking glasses handy at all times—perhaps right next to the refrigerator instead of in a cabinet. It might also mean taping a little sign to the refrigerator door that says:

HOW ABOUT
A NICE, SLENDERIZING
GLASS OF WATER?

Now, it's possible that upon self-observation and experimentation, you will not be overly impressed with the idea that you're eating in response to a hidden craving for water. Just the same, my experience in weight-control workshops suggests that making it a point to drink a lot more water is one of the smart things to do in order to promote the success of your reducing program.

Ruth said that when she came home from work every day, she would be "ravenously hungry" and immediately go to the refrigerator and begin eating. When she very consciously poured herself a glass of water immediately upon arriving home, she found that it was remarkably effective in blunting or easing her hunger pangs—which turned out to be more like impulses than true hunger. It didn't abolish the problem, but it reduced the amount she ate by a third to a half.

Carol said that going to the water fountain frequently during the day and drinking small amounts of water in the evening made her stomach feel more satisfied with less food.

The trick of success here is not to see how much water you can drink but simply to drink a few glasses. Once you do that, using very good water, you will see that it helps you, and you'll want to make it part of your daily routine.

CHAPTER

7

Dispose of Your Fat

I can see it now:

A skinny preschooler, slumped over a big wad of cold mashed potatoes. By this time, I had been playing with the potatoes so long it looked like a truck had run over them, but that didn't bother my mother a bit: "Eat those mashed potatoes! Don't you know there are children starving in Africa?"

That must have been a universal occurrence, because everyone in our diet workshop recalled a similar incident—although no one would admit playing the role of the mother in this scene!

We got a good chuckle out of that, but it wasn't so funny when I asked how many still found themselves eating just to clean their plates . . . and 11 out of 12 people raised their hands.

Eating food as an alternative to throwing it away is really a bizarre phenomenon, if you think about it.

First, as I asked the workshop participants, What do you think of the idea of using your mouth as a garbage disposal? I mean, really think about it for a minute and see how it feels.

Second, imagine the problem you face when you have a sudden and powerful impulse to put something into your mouth. Then *consider what you're doing when you shovel food into your mouth when you don't feel so much as a fleeting impulse to eat, let alone real hunger.* You may even be stuffed, but there it is, that extra piece of meat, on your plate or Susan's or Bill's, and *something* takes control of your arm and the next thing you know the food is in your mouth.

The plate is clean. Goody. And you're fat.

But just acknowledging that plate-cleaning without hunger occurs does not solve the problem, not by a long shot. Like any other habit, it needs to be worked on before it drops away. In this chapter, we're going to do that work.

First, cleaning off your plate (or someone else's) doesn't do the starving masses a lick of good.

Maybe so, you say, but isn't food *precious?* "There is something wrong with throwing food away," one person in the workshop said. "I know it may sound corny, but food is really the most valuable thing in the world and it seems like a crime to throw it away."

I can understand how someone can feel that way. Particularly if you were brought up during the Depression or the war or if you were raised in the kind of family that practically worships food. But the truth is that, although food may in fact be precious, although food may in fact be expensive, and although it does rub all of us the wrong way to see good food thrown out, *food is not scarce in the culture we live in.* Expensive, maybe, but not scarce.

Do you know the biggest single problem facing the American farmer today?

Too much food. The supply of most staples is so great that the price the farmer receives is often barely enough to pay his out-of-pocket costs. As a result of the selective breeding of dairy cows, for instance, milk production per cow has risen to the point where only the most efficient operations are able to show a respectable profit. The net result is that thousands of dairy farmers are cashing out every year. Conditions would be a lot harder for farmers if the government didn't go to great lengths to keep excess food off the market. Many people don't realize it, but the government pays "diversion" money to many farmers not to raise crops on their land, restricts the amount that other farmers are permitted to grow, and then buys up large quantities of other foodstuffs in order to keep prices at a level where most farmers can survive.

Sure, food is precious, but too much of anything can become harmful. There is no excuse, then, for eating food as an alternative to throwing it out. It's just a habit—a fattening habit.

WE ALL DO IT

Right now I want you to stop and think of some situations where you typically sweep leftovers into your mouth. Stop reading and look up at the ceiling for a minute and try to think of three situations.

We asked that question in our workshops, and here are some of the answers we got:

"When my Bobby doesn't finish what's on his plate." And how often is that? "All the time!"

"When I finish eating before my husband does, sometimes I'll sit there and keep picking, keep eating until he's done." And how often do you finish before he does? "All the time!"

"If I'm eating potato chips out of a small bag, I may be satisfied with what I've eaten, but if there're only a few left, I eat them, too. Why throw them away?" Ditto with pretzels, cookies, nuts, etc.

"If my husband pours me a beer, I'm usually filled after I drink half of it, but he says, 'Go ahead and finish it' . . . and I do."

"About once a month we go out to a restaurant and I like to order steak. It's always too much for me, but I force myself to finish it because it's so expensive."

"When we go to Mario's for pizza, it's always too much, but it's so good I hate to see it go to waste, so I help finish it off."

Here are a few other examples of compulsive plate-cleaning in action:

You open a package of three cupcakes, eat two and feel satisfied. You eat the third because it's there.

You're with friends in a restaurant and you've only eaten about half the food on your plate when you lose interest in it. But you go ahead and finish it because otherwise it will look as though you're sitting in front of a plateful of garbage.

Everybody knows that strawberry shortcake kept in the refrigerator overnight dies a slow death, and you only have one piece left, so you put it out of its misery.

In some cases, the appropriate thing to do with leftovers is to immediately wrap them and put them away. In those instances, the best thing to do is to practically jump out of your seat, wrap the food or put it in a dish and stow it.

But often there isn't enough left to be worth storing or reheating. In most cases, the only sensible thing to do is to trash it.

Before we get to actually trashing our fat, though, we're going to do a very important exercise in food consciousness. I've done it myself and so have others, and, although it may sound crazy, I assure you that it isn't. There is a real point to it. And it's fun besides.

Right now, I want you to get up, walk over to your refrigerator and open it. Now reach inside, grab some food and throw it in the trash. Go ahead, do it now. I'll wait. . . .

What did you throw out? A jar of olives that had only three or four left in the bottom? Half of a cheese sandwich three days old? Fine. How did it feel? I mean, were you nervous? Did you think you were wasting good money? Probably you felt pretty good, like cleaning house a little. I'm doing this exercise along with you, by the way, and I got off pretty easy: a plastic tube full of hot Chinese mustard.

Now I want you to go back to your refrigerator, and this time choose *two* items and throw them *both* in the trash. Really do it. This is important. . . . Well, how did you make out? Was it painful? Or was it . . . in a strange way . . . kind of fun? Personally, I enjoyed it. I took half a can of V-8 juice that had been sitting in the refrigerator for a week and poured it down the drain, and threw the can in the trash with an old and almost-used-up bottle of low-calorie salad dressing. Somehow it feels good to get old food out of the refrigerator. It doesn't belong there.

Now for the conclusion of the exercise. Go *back* to the refrigerator. This time I want you to select something that has a lot of calories in it. Pick it up, bring it to eye level, take a good look at it and imagine what all those calories would look like on your cheeks, your belly or your butt. Then say good-bye to the food . . . and *trash your fat!* Go ahead; you go to your refrigerator and I'll go to mine. I'll meet you back here in a minute.

Well, how did it feel? Terrific, right? "Liberating," was how Nick put it, describing how he had trashed three or four rich pastries that were left in a box a relative had brought over the previous day. "For the first time, I had a feeling that I was the master, not the food. . . . And it wasn't hard at all."

Just a minute ago, I had a liberating experience myself, specifically liberating a disgustingly sweet bottle of Japanese plum wine that had been sitting in my refrigerator for about a year. The funny thing is, although I *know* the techniques I'm describing here, just knowing them doesn't do you any good: You have to *practice* them. And I haven't practiced the food-liberating technique for quite a while now. Otherwise I would have realized how stupid it is to keep a horrible-tasting bottle of wine in the refrigerator indefinitely just because I paid good money (all of $2.96) for it. And having done that, I noticed that there was a bottle of off-taste eggnog that had been sitting in the back of my refrigerator since someone gave it to me at a Christmas party. That went down the drain, too.

The point of that exercise was not really to get rid of food that you would otherwise eat. I would never have consumed that wine or eggnog anyway. And perhaps you chose to sacrifice a little bit of dried-out ice cream rammed into a corner of your freezer. No matter. The idea was simply to see what it feels like to throw food away, food that you don't really want. And to realize that it isn't all that difficult. And that, perhaps, it's strangely satisfying.

The rest is easy.

FAT TRASHING IN ACTION

Now that you are fully conscious of the nature and extent of the plate-cleaning habit, and you realize that throwing away leftover food is neither sinful nor particularly difficult, you're in business. Let's say you're eating at home and the main course was spaghetti and meatballs. You've finished what was on your plate and feel quite satisfied. Not bloated, but satisfied. Little Timmy is still staring at at least half of what he started with, while your husband is finishing his second helping. In the middle of the table there is a serving dish that has one meatball in it and a little bit of spaghetti. "Go ahead and finish it off," your husband says around a mouthful of spaghetti. "It's just one meatball. And Timmy, you finish yours, too!"

Dispose of Your Fat

Being fully prepared for this potentially fattening situation, you know exactly what to do. You immediately get up, fetch the one empty custard dish in your pantry and fill it with the meatball and spaghetti that was on the serving plate. You put wrapping around it and put it in the refrigerator. "Why don't you go ahead and eat what's on Timmy's plate?" your husband suggests. You wish you could put that away, too, but there are no more empty dishes. For a second, you feel like taking your husband's advice, because you went to all the trouble of making those delicious meatballs and Timmy doesn't appreciate them. Then you suddenly realize what it is you're contemplating: *making yourself fatter because there are no available storage dishes.* Is your *stomach* a kind of storage dish? You also realize that Timmy isn't exactly starving to death and that he has in fact eaten all that his young, slender body really needs. Rather than being unappreciative, his stomach is smart enough to realize when it's had enough.

So you take away his dish and feed it to the dog. Or to the garbage can. Yes, meatball and all.

"Hey! What are you doing, throwing away a meatball?"

"Trashing my fat!"

Here's another domestic situation:

Your sister comes over to have lunch with you and your family and brings with her a large bag filled with hamburgers, milkshakes and french fries. The kids are wild about it and shout with glee. You're kind of underwhelmed by it but, when your sister brings lunch over, what are you going to do?

One thing you can do is remove the middle slice of bread from the Big Mac. Having read the chart at the back of this book, you know that a Big Mac has 540 calories, so by removing that piece of bread and some of the excess sauce from the burger, you're saving yourself about 100 calories, all of it from white bread, oil and sugar. And now the fun starts.

"What are you doing?" your sister demands. "If I had known you weren't hungry, I would have gotten you a regular hamburger!"

"Well, I do have an appetite, but it will taste just as good without the extra bread."

Your sister gives you such a look.

Five minutes later, you've polished off the burger and about three-quarters of your vanilla milkshake. Your french fries (large-size bag) are about 50 percent intact. Noticing that the kids haven't finished their milkshakes either, you take yours and spill the remainder down the drain of your sink.

"*Now* what are you doing?" your sister wants to know.

"Oh, did you want the rest of the milkshake?"

"Of course not. I have my own."

"Well, I didn't want it, either."

"A fine example you're setting for the kids!" You chuckle, but inwardly. Very inwardly.

"Anybody want more french fries?" you ask. No takers.

You roll up the bag of fries and toss it halfway across the room into the trash. Two points.

"*Are you trying to insult me?*"

"No, Sis, honest. I'm just trashing my fat!"

EAT ONLY AS MUCH AS *YOU* WANT

I've spelled these incidents out in some detail to emphasize the fact that when you begin trashing your fat, you're going to have more of a problem with other people than with yourself. Not having raised their food consciousness, as you have, they are still in the thrall of the clean-up-your-plate commandment. Handle their feelings with tact, in a very neutral way. Don't accuse them of trying to push food down your throat, even though you may sometimes feel that way. The way *they* see it, they're only being considerate.

Here is a scene at a restaurant:

Having had soup, a roll, a large salad and a glass of wine, you are ready to run up the white flag by the time you're two-thirds of the way through your expensive veal dish. For a moment you think, gee, this is nice, tender veal, and the sauce is excellent. I really ought to finish it. Then, of course, you realize how *silly* that is. All you'll be doing is *ruining* a good meal by making yourself feel bloated. So you call it quits. The problem is, being in a restaurant, you can't remove what is left, and your waiter is nowhere in sight. And if that veal just keeps sitting in front of you, you have a feeling that you are going to attack it again.

What you do is take your knife and fork and lay them across your plate in such a way that the handles become fully immersed in the sauce. Then you push your plate a few inches in front of you to signal to everyone that you're done eating, and finish off your glass of water.

Having done that, you feel quite relieved. And 10 minutes later, it's not at all difficult for you to get up and leave the table with half a glass of wine still sitting in your glass.

"Aren't you going to finish that wine?"

"I've had all I really feel like drinking." In restaurants, it's gauche to talk about trashing your fat.

Here's a particularly tricky situation:

You had dinner at the home of some new friends, and later, the hostess serves coffee and homemade pound cake. She gives you a rather large piece, and when you're halfway through it, you realize that (*a*) the pound cake isn't really that good, and (*b*) you really don't want the rest of it. What are you going to do, leave half of it on your plate? It's practically like tacking up a sign that says "This pound cake leaves something, shall we say, to be desired."

Let's backtrack a little and see if it's possible to do a little engineering. For one thing, you could have asked for a very small piece, realizing that if the pound cake proved to be especially good, your hostess would ask you if you wanted more, and you could flatter her by saying "Yes, it's delicious!"

Now, in this particular case, she didn't ask you what size piece you wanted, so upon being handed the large slice, you could have said "Oh, I know I'll never be able to finish this!"

"Really? Are you still full from dinner?"

"Well, I just feel very *comfortable* right now, and lately my stomach seems to have shrunk."

So if you decide not to finish it, no one is going to be surprised or insulted.

But let's assume that you didn't do either of these things and you're just sitting there looking at a couple of hundred calories' worth of insipid cake. Or maybe it really is good, but you just don't feel like finishing it anyway. What you do in a situation like that is to quickly put up a "sign" of your own. "Mrs. Smith, I'm sorry that I have to waste part of your cake, but pound cake is so rich. It fills me up really fast."

Now you *could* say "Gee, Mrs. Smith, this pound cake is really *fabulous* but blah blah blah," but I wouldn't recommend that. If the cake is not really good, your hostess will almost certainly realize it and either think you're a liar or tell you so to your face: "You don't have to make excuses; this is a lousy recipe."

My advice is to be tactful but honest. That is a good combination in many situations.

CHAPTER

8

Mealtime Strategies That Make Dieting Unnecessary

How many times have you gotten up from the dinner table with the feeling that you ate more than you really wanted—perhaps just a *little* too much, but just enough to make you feel uncomfortably full?

If that feeling of being stuffed to the gills is a familiar one, you need to restructure your mealtime eating habits.

If you usually feel satisfied but not stuffed—except after a holiday feast—mealtime probably isn't your problem.

On the other hand, if you seldom feel really satisfied after eating a meal, you probably *do* have a major mealtime problem—one that might be worse than feeling stuffed, because it's increasing the likelihood of late-night binges.

You might think that the purely subjective feeling you have upon getting up from the table is a poor way to judge whether or not you have eaten too much, but in truth it's probably the best way. The idea that someone on a reducing diet ought to eat a dinner consisting of precisely 500 or 700 calories is simply ridiculous. Why should a 220-pound man be satisfied or nourished by the same meal prescribed for a 165-pound man? Yet that is the approach traditionally taken in diet plans, and it is another reason why they almost always fail.

The most important thing to understand about dinnertime, I think, is that eating a meal is a *ritual,* perhaps the most basic ritual of human life. It's something you have done tens of thousands of times. Each of us brings to the occasion all sorts of deeply ingrained habits and expectations. For many of us, dinnertime is also an important social occasion. It may be the only time that the family gets together as a unit to share an activity. If that's the case, anger or frustration that may have been building all day may suddenly erupt at the table. Likewise, feelings of friendship and love that may be bottled up during the rest of the day may suddenly find expression over meat and potatoes.

The moral is that if we pretend dinnertime is nothing but shoveling food into our mouths in a kind of social vacuum, all that energy endemic to the mealtime ritual is going to rapidly overwhelm our best intentions and drown them in a bowl of gravy. But if we understand something about that ritualistic energy and plan our changes accordingly, we may discover that it really isn't that difficult to achieve success—right from the very first day.

Mealtime actually begins long before somebody says, "Dinner is ready!" Let's consider the following true example.

Julia summons her husband and children to the table. The main course is scallops, which both Julia and her husband enjoy greatly. But trouble starts fast. Because scallops were so expensive, Julia was able to buy only a small amount. As soon as her husband sees the skimpy portion on his plate, he gets a frustrated feeling and lets Julia know about it. That makes Julia feel very distressed, so she immediately goes to the refrigerator and comes back with all sorts of leftovers, which she piles in front of her husband as a kind of testimony to the fact that she still loves him. She also gives her husband several of her scallops, which gives *her* a ticket to dive into the leftovers, too. Twenty minutes later, both of their stomachs are bursting with scallops, vegetables, potato salad and cold beef sandwiches. Still trying to make up for a botched meal, Julia gives her husband an especially large helping of dessert. And to make herself feel better, she has some extra pie, too . . . only instead of feeling better, she feels worse.

There are innumerable variations on that theme. But what they all boil down to is that the unstructured meal easily becomes an occasion to plunder the refrigerator and pillage the pantry in a desperate attempt to put something on the table that is going to feel like dinner. Almost invariably, it's a case of overkill. And "kill" is probably the right word. Because what we're doing amounts to killing the appetite by brute force rather than satisfying it with the kind of careful, loving attention our bodies deserve.

A disorganized meal is bad not only because it can lead to too much food being put on the table. When there is no structure or "theme" to a meal, it actually takes more food, more calories, to give us that sense of satisfaction we desire. Recall how much you had to eat to feel satisfied the last time you had a really fine and attractively served meal. Compare that to the amount you had to eat to reach satisfaction the last time you sat down (or stood up) to a chaotic kind of potluck meal. Somehow, if it doesn't seem like a "real dinner," you may find yourself eating excessive amounts of food simply to convince yourself that you really *had* dinner.

LEARN TO STRUCTURE YOUR MEAL

Our first principle, then, is: *Always know what you're going to have for dinner well before you begin preparing a meal.* If you get into the habit of doing that, there will be no pressing need to measure portions, count calories or forgo your favorite foods. When you plan your meals, eating appropriate portions will follow naturally.

Planning a meal begins at the kitchen table—not with knife and fork but with pencil and paper. For most people, planning meals about a week in advance works best. Whether you're going to be trying some new recipes, relying on family favorites, or both, it's extremely helpful to have the actual list of ingredients right in front of you. It's worth double-checking to make sure that you have all the appropriate condiments for each recipe or meal: Parmesan cheese for the pasta, lemon for the fish, yogurt for the baked potato and so forth. Herbs, spices and condiments help give food the quality of being a "meal," which is exactly the quality that we're striving for.

Principle Number Two: *Try to buy only as much food as will fit into your planned menus.* There are two ways to do this. One is to make every effort not to buy excessive amounts of food in the first place, and the other is to learn how to use leftovers in a creative but planned manner. If you're the kind of person who knows how to turn leftovers into a good lunch or dinner, you have a definite advantage here. If not, you can either ask friends for tips, buy some recipe books or be especially diligent when making your purchases. That may mean, for instance, going a little out of your way to buy meat from a butcher instead of the supermarket, in order to get the portions you really want. Instead of buying a whole chicken, you may want to buy a couple of split breasts or some legs. A butcher will usually give you exactly the amount of ground beef you want, and it's easy to store leftovers, raw or cooked, for future use. You may also want to emphasize nonmeat items—rice, bulgur, noodles, beans and potatoes—in your diet, because many are easily stored and conveniently portioned.

It's interesting that just as the easily stored and portioned foods mentioned above are high in nutrition and low in fat, foods that can create real leftover problems tend to be high in fat or calories: pork roasts, spareribs and all sorts of cakes, pies and special desserts. The biggest trouble with a chocolate cake, for instance, is not so much the calories in one piece but the difficulty so many of us have in keeping the leftover portion for later use. That "later use" too often turns out to be 3 hours after you've had your first serving.

Principle Number Three: *Don't put more on the table than you want to eat at that meal.* In the case of the chocolate cake mentioned before, the sensible thing to do is to cut out one large piece that can be divided into a reasonable portion for everyone at the table and then wrap and store the remainder. Putting the rest of that cake in the freezer may also be a good idea, so you won't have to "worry" that it will go bad unless you polish it off. Some cooks enjoy bringing a large roast or casserole to the table because it looks very impressive. But if experience tells you that all that food sitting on the table is going to create a desire to eat more than you really want, do the carving or serving on the kitchen countertop and then store the rest before eating. An alternative would be to put the whole dish on the table, serve the food, then immediately remove what's left and store it. If you're really hungry, you can always get more, and there's nothing at all wrong with doing that. *All you're trying to do is structure your dinner in such a way as to encourage a pattern of eating based on real hunger, instead of habit, impulse and the plate-cleaning syndrome.* Remember: Food that is sitting on the table during a meal is more likely to be consumed "unconsciously" than in any other situation.

Principle Number Four: *Take away leftovers and unfinished dinners as soon as possible, for storage or disposal.* This principle is simply the follow-through to the previous one. If there's anything more apt to be eaten unconsciously than extra food sitting on the table at dinnertime, it's extra food sitting on your *plate* after you've finished your main bout of eating. Somehow there's always that extra potato, a few extra tablespoons of gravy, that piece of bread or half of Jimmy's dinner that mysteriously winds up on your own plate. The place for that extra food is the refrigerator, the bread box—or the garbage can, if need be. If it feels like it's a shame not to "do something" with that good food, just stop for a moment and picture what that "good food" is going to look like on your neck and thighs. Do you really want to use your body as a kind of warehouse or silo? If not, get busy and clean off that table!

SIDETRACK YOUR EATING MOMENTUM

The fifth and last principle is really a comprehensive set of skills that I call *learning to sidetrack your eating momentum.*

Through observation of my own eating habits and questioning of workshop participants, it became clear to me that a considerable amount of overeating that takes place at dinnertime is the result of an almost mindless momentum. This momentum builds up rapidly and doesn't grind to a halt until you've eaten *much* more than you need, *considerably* more than you really wanted and just enough to make you feel like every cell in your body has been stuffed full of food. Many of us, I'm sure, astonish ourselves with our ability to eat large bowls of soup, buttered rolls, heaping plates of salad and big chunks of meat without putting the brakes on that momentum. Often that eating drive doesn't sputter to a halt until we sneak pieces of food from serving dishes even as we carry them to the refrigerator to be stored.

Yet, 15 minutes later, we feel so overfed that we realize it wasn't true hunger that made us eat all that extra food. It was nothing but sheer *eating momentum.*

The most dangerous—and ineffective—way to stop something with a lot of momentum behind it, whether it's a locomotive or your appetite, is to stand in front of it and let it plow into you. When we do that with a locomotive, it's called suicide; when we do it with eating momentum, it's called willpower.

The right way, the effective way, of reducing the dangerous momentum from an onrushing object is to sidetrack it, divert its energy off on a tangent, a safe tangent, where it can either run out of steam naturally or be braked in a variety of ways until it reaches a manageable energy level.

What that means at the dinner table is that rather than merely giving ourselves small portions of food and then jumping up from the table in a spasm of willpower, we're going to reengineer our dinner ritual, lay down some new tracks as it were, so that we can control the momentum that keeps us eating past the point where we've had enough.

The single, most important cause of uncontrollable eating momentum is the failure of our nervous systems to throw our appetites into neutral when our stomachs have received an appropriate amount of food. How often have you finished eating, not feeling particularly stuffed, only to feel positively sluggish and bloated 20 or 30 minutes later? That's the failure I'm referring to, although "failure" might not be the right word.

It would be nice, wouldn't it, if our stomachs and the nerve centers with which they communicate could give us what computer people call "real-time feedback" a few seconds after we swallow each morsel of food. That way, we would know—*and feel*—exactly how far along we were in the process of meeting our metabolic needs, and when they were satisfied, our appetites would instantly and automatically be thrown into neutral.

But as we all know, that doesn't happen. And for good reason. Our eating control system, by which I refer to the whole complex of organs, nerves and chemical substances that regulate appetite, is too smart to be caught playing that instant feedback game. Were it to do that, we would probably all be stumbling around in a state of severe malnutrition, because every time we ate a few pieces of fruit or some bulky, low-calorie vegetables or drank two glasses of water, we'd feel as though we'd just eaten a complete meal.

What our appetite control system wants to do before signaling us that it's time to quit is *analyze* what we've eaten and find out if it contains enough real nourishment. And that takes some time, because food first has to be processed by stomach acids, move through the pyloric valve into the small intestine and then be absorbed—at least partially—into the system. At that point, the control system knows what we've eaten and is prepared to begin downshifting our jaw muscles. Scientists who have studied this process say that it takes about 20 to 25 minutes for it to occur—and those 20 minutes become a critical factor in learning to sidetrack your eating momentum.

Actually, some people, particularly children and very slender adults, seem to respond to food more quickly than that and experience the sensation of fullness within 5 or 10 minutes after they begin eating. My belief is that that greater sensitivity is a natural gift many of us lose—along with other natural sensitivities—as we grow older and become accustomed to responding more to external cues than to our own bodies and spirits. In fact, it's my experience that as you begin to control your eating and begin slowly to lose weight, some of that sensitivity returns. If after dieting for a while, you've said that "my stomach seems to have shrunk," what you're experiencing, I believe, is the return of that sensitivity.

But until such time as your appetite control system may learn to respond more quickly, you have to live with the reality of that 20-minute delay.

How to slow down.   Many if not most people who eat too much at a meal also eat too rapidly. Naturally, the more quickly you eat, the more you can put away before your appetite control system has a chance to swing into action. There is also a psychological component here, because many people who eat too rapidly are barely conscious that they're eating. Their attention is focused on a newspaper or a heavy conversation. Many people eat while they're watching TV. Since your brain is an integral part of your appetite control system, why not let it in on the fact that you're eating dinner?

Just *how* slowly you ought to eat is difficult to say. Probably the best thing to do is experiment with various speeds. You can begin by trying to eat about 50 percent more slowly than you do now—assuming that you're a fast eater. First tell yourself, "I'm going to eat dinner now." Then look at the food on your plate very carefully. Describe it to yourself. When you take your first bite of something, put down your silverware and chew your food slowly and thoroughly, so that you experience its flavor, texture and aroma. Take another forkful of food only after you have thoroughly savored and swallowed your first. Put down your silverware again, lean back in your chair and enjoy yourself. *Be aware that eating is one of the most important things you do and that it's perfectly reasonable to eat in a slow and thoughtful manner.* Most people also find eating quite enjoyable, so why eat as fast as you can? Your new way of eating will not only make the experience last longer, it will also make it more enjoyable because you'll be much more in touch with the experience of eating—as opposed to unconsciously shoveling food into your mouth.

If you want to, you can experiment with techniques that *really* slow down eating. If you're right-handed, hold your fork in your left hand. Chew each mouthful of food 50 times. Wait 15 seconds between mouthfuls. Try chewing your food in slow motion, as if it were the last morsel of food you were ever going to have in your life. If dinner comes in different courses, try waiting 5 minutes between courses. Or plan your meal so that it's served that way. In between courses, get up from the table and prepare the next course, or do something else. Don't keep sitting at the table, or you'll become terribly impatient.

Some of these techniques may sound a little unnatural, but I'm not so sure they are. I vividly remember watching a big Siberian tiger at the Philadelphia Zoo just before feeding time. When the feeding man came in with a can of raw meat, all the big cats began to growl and leap around their cages. Finally it was the tiger's turn to be thrown a big chunk of horse meat. I expected him to swallow the thing practically whole. But just the opposite happened. He picked up his dinner in his jaws, walked over to the middle of his cage, eased himself down into a comfortable position and proceeded to make love to that hunk of horse meat. He licked it, nibbled it, sniffed it and finally began chewing it, very slowly, in the corner of his mouth. Now there's somebody who *enjoys* his dinner!

I confess I don't lick my meat, but if eating like that is good enough for a Siberian tiger, it can't be all that unnatural.

Another technique that can help slow down your eating momentum is to change the *time* that you eat dinner. Many of our workshop participants said that if they ate immediately upon coming home from work, their appetites seemed to be particularly ravenous. Ironically, several said that if they waited an hour or two to have dinner, they felt much less hungry. That may not seem to make much sense, but if you think about it, you may find that when you return from a day's work, your "appetite" at that moment is being fueled by tension built up during the day and probably the tension involved in driving home. What seems to be happening is that as soon as you leave work, you know that the next thing on the agenda is to eat, and expectation of that meal keeps building up until you get to the kitchen. Often, the eagerness to eat is so great that you begin eating within seconds of entering your house. But what's driving you at that moment is not true hunger but a pattern of habit, expectation and tension.

One of our workshop participants had the same experience I did: When she delayed dinner for about 2 hours—filling that time with carefully planned activities such as a walk and household chores—she found that her hunger had greatly abated. Although you may never have tried that technique, you may have experienced the results just the same. Did you ever "lose your appetite" because a meal habitually eaten at a certain time was delayed for half an hour or more? If your motive was purely hunger, that wouldn't happen. The edge was taken off your appetite simply because a long-standing habit pattern had suddenly been broken.

A variation of that approach is to try making lunch your main meal instead of dinner. For the last few months, that's what I've been doing, and it seems to be working well. Because I eat lunch out, there is no opportunity to raid the pantry. Then, at dinnertime, I have something light, like melon and cottage cheese. (On this regimen, I discovered that my energy level for evening work maintained a much more even keel.)

No matter how large their dinner, many people still have a desire for something sweet before leaving the table. That is nothing more than sheer habit, like wanting a cigarette after a meal, and with a little effort, the desire will abate. By eating a large salad at the end of your meal, most of the battle will be won, because habitually you don't eat sweets right after a salad. There may also be something to the theory that strongly flavored foods like meats and rich sauces encourage the desire for something sweet immediately afterward, to balance the taste buds, perhaps. Finishing the meal with something relatively bland, like salad or even some bread, will help.

What works for me is a cup of unsweetened peppermint tea, which also leaves the mouth feeling clean and satisfied. If you like an occasional cup of tea or coffee, it's a good idea to have one already brewed and waiting so that you can immediately enjoy it when you're done eating. You will find that in a short time you will lay down a new habit pattern, so that the drinking of your tea becomes a powerful signaling device to your system that the meal has come to a conclusion.

However you conclude your meal, you should tell yourself: "This is the way I'm *supposed* to feel. Not stuffed, but satisfied. This feeling is really much better than being stuffed and sluggish. Fifteen minutes from now I'll feel even more satisfied than I am now. So why should I clog up my body's machinery with too much food?"

At that point, leave the table and immediately begin some purposeful activity. Whether it's washing the dishes or reading a book, taking your dog for a walk or sewing, the idea is that you should *know* what you're going to do, so that you don't simply sit at the table for lack of anything better to do.

If others are still at the table and you want to enjoy their company, take away your own plate, wash your hands and then return to the table. Or carry on a conversation while you do the dishes at the sink. One of the best techniques is to return to the table with some knitting, because no one is going to eat unconsciously while knitting. If you enjoy playing a musical instrument, right after dinner is a fine time to practice. An evening chess game immediately after dinner, right at the cleaned-off table, is another good idea.

Modifications in mealtime behavior are a process of trial and error, of experimentation, of self-discovery and of health improvement. Expect that many of the things you try will not work out exactly right. But learn from them. It may take weeks or even months until you feel comfortable with a new set of mealtime eating habits. But keep trying— not with your willpower, but with your thinking, planning and experimenting. Those are the tools that are going to work for you.

9

The 300 Plan for Painless Calorie Cutting

We haven't said much so far about calories per se. That's because I wanted to emphasize the fact that the path to success is not so much a way of dieting as a way of eating. A new, more natural and healthful way of eating that will let you lose weight, yes, but much more important, maintain your ideal weight once you have reached it.

Having made this point, it's now time to talk about calories and what they mean. Doing so will enable you to visualize the effect that changes in eating habits are going to have on your waistline. We will also take advantage of this discussion of calories to review some of the eating techniques we've already learned and to introduce some new ones.

I suppose the most basic fact is that when you eat 3,000 calories that are not burned up by your metabolic needs or exercise, you will gain 1 pound of fat. Perhaps you have read that the consumption of 3,500 calories is required to create 1 pound of fat. That's the figure that is generally used. But like so much else that's published about weight control, even that simple statement is wrong. It's true that

3,500 calories can lead to the formation of 1 pound of fat, but only *theoretically*. Because as soon as you begin depositing fat in your body, you begin to retain water. Even the cells in which the fat is enveloped have to gain weight to take care of the extra burden. The result is that—largely because of water retention—you only have to consume about 2,950 calories to add 1 pound of excess weight to your body. For the sake of convenience, let's say 3,000 calories.

If you overeat by 100 calories a day, then, you will gain 1 pound in about 30 days.

If you eat 100 calories *less* than you require to meet your needs, you will *lose* 1 pound in the same amount of time.

But suppose you go on eating 100 calories a day less than your current requirements for a whole year. Will you lose 12 pounds? Would you lose 24 pounds in 2 years? Would you lose 240 pounds in 20 years and vanish from the face of the earth? Thankfully, no. Weight loss doesn't work that way.

When you have lost 1 extra pound of fat, you have at that point decreased the number of calories you are automatically burning up each day by about 10. That's the approximate number of calories that were required to keep that pound of fat at body temperature, care for its metabolic needs and carry it around all day. When you have lost 10 pounds, you will be burning up about 100 calories less each day than you were when you were heavier. So, at that point, the 100-calorie dent you put in your diet will no longer have any effect. You'll be 10 pounds lighter and stay that way—as long as your diet doesn't change. But put those 100 calories back, and the 10 pounds will follow like chubby little sheep.

That explains why the pattern of weight loss is usually to drop weight relatively quickly in the early stages, then progressively more slowly. As the pounds fall away, your requirement for food drops and your dieting has a less dramatic effect.

It works the same way with exercise. If you begin burning up 100 calories more each day than you have been and keep your calorie intake the same, you will eventually drop 10 pounds. At that point, you'll stop losing weight. Let's say you weighed 160 when you began your moderate exercise program. Now you weigh just 150, and your need for calories is less. And that lesser amount you're burning up at your slimmer weight is 100 calories—or exactly what you're spending in exercise. You've arrived at equilibrium. If you want to lose further, you either have to eat less—in keeping with your smaller frame—or exercise more.

We can turn this around, too, and see why overeating doesn't usually turn us into blimps. If you're eating, say, 200 calories more than your body size and exercise habits require to maintain equilibrium, you will eventually gain about 20 pounds. But no more. Because the 20 pounds you put on will be "eating" those 200 calories. Cutting back on exercise works the same way. Stop your habitual exercise which burned up 200 calories a day and you'll eventually add 20 pounds—and stay there.

The math may not work out exactly in real life, but the principle does. You may find, for instance, that cutting 100 calories a day out of your diet only produces a loss of 7 or 8 pounds, not 10. Not all of us have the same basal metabolic rate—the number of calories we burn up per pound just to stay alive. But the principle holds up. When you reduce your food intake (or begin exercising), the weight loss you experience will be faster in the beginning, and will slow down considerably as the months go by. It's important to realize that *this is perfectly natural*. Don't get discouraged if weight loss in your third month is noticeably slower than in the first. It *has* to be that way. If it wasn't, even a slight reduction in calories would eventually turn you into a skeleton!

Of course, you can always make a further reduction in daily calories if things seem to be slowing up too much. Just use common sense. If you need to lose only 15 pounds, there is no point in cutting 500 calories from your daily diet. But if you need to lose 60 pounds, realize that even 500 calories won't get you there. The best technique is probably to cut back in stages. When you get used to eating 300 calories a day less, for instance, go for 400. Hold there for a month or two, and then trim more.

THE 300 PLAN

Which brings us to a question that eventually comes up for some readers. Namely, just *how many* calories is it reasonable to remove from your diet?

"I've been following your approach and becoming more conscious of how and why I'm eating," Warren said. "But I feel a little uneasy about it because I'm not really sure if what I'm cutting out of my diet is a reasonable amount. Maybe it's even too much."

For people like Warren, who feel more comfortable with some additional guidance, I have come up with what I call the 300 Plan. This plan suggests that 300 calories a day is a good average figure of calorie reduction to aim for, at least during the first few months of reducing. It also helps locate the most "vulnerable" 300 calories in a diet and then suggests ways by which they can be done away with in a relatively harmless fashion.

Some people do not need this guidance, and there is nothing terribly special about the figure of 300 calories. I have chosen that as an average figure to aim for because experience shows that most people can cut that much out of their daily food intake without feeling hungry, deprived or weak. It's also enough of a reduction to produce a loss of 30 pounds. However, my advice is to *combine* this cutback of 300 calories of food with an *increase* of about 200 calories worth of exercise—equivalent to about 45 minutes of easy walking. That combined approach will produce a deficit of some 500 calories a day, producing a weight loss of about 5 pounds the first month and slightly but progressively less each succeeding month, with the net effect being a loss of 50 pounds.

If you need to lose only about 25 pounds, it will be easy (lucky you!) to simply change the 300 Plan to a 150 Plan. But the principle and techniques will be the same.

What if you want to lose *more* than 50 pounds? What then? That's a good question, and as a matter of fact it came up when I contacted a young woman who was one of the more diligent members of one of the workshops. By the end of the workshop, she said, she had lost exactly 45 pounds by changing her eating behavior and walking daily. She also said she has had "no trouble" keeping that weight off. However, she hasn't been able to lose any more weight, and she still wants to lose about another 20 pounds. She was puzzled, too, because she didn't understand why her weight loss didn't continue.

I explained to her that having lost 45 pounds, she was now burning some 450 calories a day less than she was when she began the program. In other words, she had reached the point at which less food and more exercise (amounting to 450 calories a day) were exactly balancing the caloric needs of her new, lower weight.

I went on to advise her that she should be very aware of the fact that she is now, very literally, *a new person*. That while a reduction of 300 calories a day was appropriate for her a year ago, her needs are so much smaller now, and her true hunger so much less, that it would be not only appropriate but relatively easy to decrease her caloric input still more. I suggested that she reduce her daily calorie total by another 100 calories a day. At the same time, I suggested she try for more exercise, which would burn up about another 100 calories a day. (In fact, she'd just joined a health spa.) Following that plan, the last 20 pounds of her unwanted fat would inevitably fall away.

It's easy to modify the principles of the 300 Plan so that it *eventually* becomes a 400 Plan or a 500 Plan. Remember, after losing 30 pounds on the 300 Plan (or more if you're exercising), you have become a new person. It is perfectly reasonable and logical for you to cut back your food intake at that point. And to keep reducing it, *gradually,* until you reach the point where you are at your ideal weight and your losing has come to a natural end.

And what happens at that point? Nothing! You just keep on doing exactly as you have been, following your new habits. There is no "diet" to go off. You completely avoid the trap that destroys people who lose a lot of weight following a 1,200-calorie diet and then, when they reach their target weight, simply revert to eating the way they were before. Instead, you change nothing, realizing that you have engineered for yourself a new way of eating and living that is perfectly designed to maintain your ideal weight.

It may have struck you that weight loss in this approach is not produced at blinding speed. But that's a plus, not a minus. Any expert in weight reduction will tell you that the more quickly weight comes off, the more quickly it comes back. Both your body and your behavior *need* that time in order to become totally accustomed to new eating patterns. So, although it may sound a little strange, it's important to realize that *it is better to lose weight slowly than rapidly.* We already know that our problem is not losing weight, anyway, but keeping it off, and your chances of maintaining your new weight will be enormously greater if you lose your weight over a period of, say, one year, rather than three months.

You will be much better off aiming for a very modest reduction of calories at first and then gradually increasing it, rather than aiming for too great an initial decrease. If there is any optimal rate of weight loss, my estimate is that it would be in the vicinity of 3 pounds a month if you're doing it by reduced food intake alone and about 5 pounds a month if you're combining the dietary approach with exercise. *That means a weight reduction of anywhere between 36 and 60 pounds in a year's time.* More important, it means weight reduction that's much more likely to be *permanent.*

THE 300 PLAN IN ACTION

Now let's see what removing 300 calories a day actually looks like and feels like.

Keep in mind that the foods I am listing here are those which are habitually or typically part of your daily diet and that you are *not* going to eat.

The second important point is that the foods selected for these daily deductions are chosen not simply because they happen to add up to 300 calories but also because they fall into one or more of the following categories.

- Junk foods that contribute nothing to your well-being.
- Foods that are typically consumed as snacks (recreational eating).
- Foods that can be divided in such a way that you can eat less of them without feeling deprived.
- Foods that are consumed as second helpings (often because of the sheer momentum of rapid eating or permitting them to sit on the table after the meal has been completed).
- Foods that don't give you a great sense of satisfaction.

	Calories
One-half cup beef hash	200
One can ginger ale	113
Total	313

In the first example, the half-cup of beef hash represents a second helping that is habitually eaten but is now not even put on the table. The can of ginger ale, consumed largely for its amusement value, has been pushed out of the picture by good spring water, club soda or coffee. Even if a teaspoon of sugar were added to the coffee, the total saving for the day would still be 300 calories.

	Calories
One-half piece buttered toast w/jelly	70
One tablespoon Russian dressing	75
One Coke	144
One very small cheese cracker (145 per pound)	15
Total	304

This example, like most of the others we'll be giving, is arranged in the approximate order that these food items typically appear in the daily diet. Let's say that this individual typically breakfasts on a glass of orange juice, one scrambled egg, one piece of buttered toast with jelly, and a cup of coffee. He decides to try eating half of that piece of toast and discovers that he can do it without feeling hungry or deprived. He might have left off the jelly and eaten the entire piece of buttered toast and saved almost as many calories, but when he tried that, he found that without the jelly, he *did* feel unsatisfied.

He then went on to eat his usual lunch, but at dinner, when he typically used 2 tablespoons of Russian dressing on his salad, he cut out one of those tablespoons by the simple expedient of tossing the salad with the dressing in a big bowl. After dinner, he typically would have a bottle of Coke and a handful of cheese crackers; now he has half a cup of coffee and one or two fewer cheese crackers. And he's very careful about not eating those crackers from the box but rather removing the exact number that he wants to eat and then putting the box in the back of the pantry.

	Calories
One-half tablespoon mayonnaise	50
Five potato chips	55
One pat butter	36
One-third cup pork and beans	104
One dozen shelled, roasted peanuts	60
Total	305

This man hasn't changed his breakfast. His first deduction comes at lunch, when he tells the waiter at his favorite restaurant that he'd like the cook to go easy on the mayonnaise on his turkey sandwich and to hold the potato chips. At dinner, he spreads only a little butter on his bread and his vegetables (using prewarmed butter that will spread thinly) and forgoes the second helping of pork and beans. Later, at 9:00, he skips his usual handful of salted nuts.

	Calories
One-half piece buttered toast	55
One large forkful apple pie	50
Two thin pretzels	70
One slice pizza	153
Total	328

Sally lives with family members who typically have pie after almost every meal. Although she "doesn't eat any herself," she does take one forkful, which "can't hurt." She finds out that it *does* hurt when she does it three times a week, and she gives up this habit. It so happens that this is a Friday night, when she and her husband typically go out and split a pizza. Usually her husband will have five pieces, while she has three. After thinking about it, she realizes that after eating two, she's perfectly satisfied and that, in fact, that third piece makes her feel uncomfortable. So she decides to "trash her fat" and leave the piece on the pizza pan whether her husband eats it or not.

	Calories
One slice bacon	43
Two cheese/peanut butter cracker "sandwiches"	70
Three large prunes	60
One-half cup Jell-O	71
Six cashews	68
Total	312

This woman eats a fairly substantial breakfast, so one less slice of bacon isn't going to interfere seriously with her normal eating pattern. After that, she accomplishes everything she needs to in the way of calorie reduction simply by removing a few snacks. Notice, incidentally, how many calories there are in a couple of peanut-butter-and-cheese crackers!

	Calories
One-half cup coleslaw (made w/mayonnaise)	85
One slice American cheese	105
One piece bologna	57
One-quarter cup ice cream	64
One rye wafer	20
Total	331

Here's a person who does not eat a great deal of junk food or even many desserts, except for a half-cup of ice cream every night at about 11:00. Most of the overeating seems to be in the afternoon. The deductions came with the simple expedients of a serving of coleslaw only half as large as usual and eating a sandwich made with only one piece of cheese and two pieces of bologna rather than two pieces of cheese and three pieces of bologna. Then, at night, she still had the ice cream snack, but cut the portion in half.

	Calories
One slice baked ham (4 in. × 4 in.)	50
One-half slice Swiss cheese (4 in. × 4 in.)	65
One-half hard roll	78
Five ounces beer	63
One-quarter cup buttered noodles	60
Total	316

This example is a variation on the previous one and shows how flexibility and experimentation will lead you to discover the most effective way for you to cut down your caloric overshoot without making yourself feel deprived. Walter does not feel satisfied unless the sandwich he is eating has a certain *thickness* to it, so he kept that the same, or even a bit bigger than before, except that now he is eating only *half* a sandwich.

But what's this business about 5 ounces of beer? No, I'm not going to ask you to pour the second half of that bottle of beer down the drain. Those 5 ounces of beer are what you don't drink if, instead of buying your beer in the usual 12-ounce bottle, you buy it by the pony, which contains only 7 ounces. True, not every brand comes in the pony size, but there's precious little difference between one brand of beer and another anyway. At least American beer.

	Calories
One-half corned beef sandwich	175
One-third tablespoon salad oil	40
One Oreo cookie	50
One fig bar cookie	50
Total	315

The big deduction here comes from eliminating half of a corned beef sandwich, which for this person is a typical Saturday night after-theater snack. What she did was convince her husband to split the sandwich with her rather than each ordering a whole one. They discovered that half a sandwich is quite enough to satisfy them. The reduction in the salad oil is gained by the simple expedient of tossing the salad more. And the two cookies represent the elimination of some "amusement" eating.

	Calories
One-half sausage link	35
One-half buttered pancake with syrup	90
Two saltines	24
One beer	151
Total	300

Here's another example of reducing by sharing. The husband and wife each typically had one sausage link and two pancakes for breakfast each day. Now they cook only one link and share it, and instead of grilling four pancakes, they make only three, sharing the third one. At dinnertime, this person eats two saltines instead of the usual four, and she has decided that she is going to cut out her nightly beer on Monday through Thursday evenings.

	Calories
One Coke	144
One-quarter cup creamed chipped beef	95
Two small chocolate-coated mints	90
Total	329

If you put all this food together, it wouldn't look like much, but when you overeat by this much every day, it does look like a lot when it builds up on your hips! That Coke could easily be replaced by water, club soda or coffee. The small amount of creamed chipped beef is a second helping not taken, or perhaps a slightly smaller first helping. The two mints are typical examples of an "amusement" snack.

	Calories
One root beer	152
One piece Boston brown bread w/cream cheese	155
Total	307

Here is a good illustration of how a person who habitually eats a number of snack foods each day can accomplish the desired reduction by eliminating just two items. Two more "deuces" follow.

		Calories
Two cups buttered popcorn		82
Four graham crackers		220
	Total	302

		Calories
One Twinkie		190
One cup Hawaiian Punch		110
	Total	300

Three-quarters cup chocolate pudding	290 calories

And sometimes, as in this example and those below, the elimination of just *one* snack (which is eaten habitually) can achieve the desired reduction.

One piece marble cake	290 calories
One hot dog on roll	295 calories
One piece cherry pie	308 calories
One Hostess fruit pie	460 calories

These single deductions seem to be letting the person off easy, but keep in mind that anyone who eats cake *every day* may be considerably overweight. In that case, it would be appropriate to increase the daily deductions, after about two months, to 400 calories a day.

Sometimes it's not a single item but a single "assault" on a box or can or tray of snacks that can account for the sum of your daily caloric overshoot, and then some. For instance:

Six fig bar cookies	300 calories
Two Ring Dings	320 calories
Six oatmeal-raisin cookies	354 calories

Sometimes the solution can be found in the elimination of one or two items, not ordinarily thought of as especially fattening, that are nibbled throughout the day. For instance:

		Calories
Fifteen very small cheese crackers		225
Five teaspoons sugar		75
	Total	300

The 300 Plan for Painless Calorie Cutting

In this example, the person typically drank about six cups of coffee a day. She found that she was able to learn to enjoy her coffee without sugar, except for the first cup of the day.

Some people who eat "health foods" almost exclusively find themselves overweight despite their avoidance of junk food. You can get some idea of why that may be so from looking at the next three examples.

		Calories
Three medium figs		120
One-half cup grape juice		83
Five large prunes		100
	Total	303

		Calories
Five dates		110
One-quarter cup dried peach halves		105
One tablespoon honey		64
Three unshelled peanuts		30
	Total	309

		Calories
Six walnuts		158
Six roasted almonds		46
Three Brazil nuts		93
	Total	297

As you can see at a glance, dried fruits and nuts (seeds, too) are not only nutritional gold mines but caloric gold mines as well. It's one thing to eat them as part of the food you actually require—in fact, that's an excellent idea. But when you eat too much of these concentrated foods, the results quickly become obvious.

There are even some fresh fruits, popular among health food people, that pack a caloric wallop:

		Calories
One mango		152
One-half avocado		188
	Total	340

Notice the caloric density of just half an avocado and keep it in mind the next time you think of making an avocado dip (guacamole).

While ordinarily you will be deducting foods eaten at a number of times throughout the day, it's quite possible that the elimination of just one snack time can turn the tide for you.

	Calories
One cherry soda	171
Six thin pretzels	140
Total	311

Here's a teenager who, on returning from school each day, sits down in front of the TV and has a soda and a handful of pretzels. That may not sound like much, but it adds up. And sitting in front of the TV makes matters worse. In this case, the elimination of that one snack—which is accomplished by going out for 30 minutes of walking—was quite sufficient to achieve the desired weight loss and control.

Here's another example of a single snacking session, repeated on a daily basis, or close to it, that, if eliminated, would be sufficient to achieve a respectable weight loss:

	Calories
Three and one-half ounces white wine	87
One ounce cheddar cheese	113
Five rye wafers	100
Total	300

This example brings up an important point. *In deciding what you are not going to eat, it is vital to know what you can give up without feeling deprived and what you can't. To discover this may require repeated experimentation.*

For instance, in the example above, it's possible that the wine, cheese and rye wafers don't represent merely so many calories, but a daily ritual that has come to be an important part of that person's life. It's something he looks forward to, something that helps him relax at the end of the workday. If he enjoys it with his wife, it may also be an important social or domestic event. If all that is the case, and the entire snack consists of what is listed above, you can imagine that simply whipping it out of the daily diet is going to create a troublesome vacuum. Of course, there are an infinite number of ways to fill that vacuum, including a shared walk, a shared hobby activity or perhaps starting right in to make dinner together. *But that vacuum must be filled somehow.*

There's also the possibility that the food listed above consists of only *half* the wine and cheese consumed and that halving the snack is not going to cause any feeling of deprivation.

Another possibility would be to modify the snack somewhat. For instance, along with the wine, each person might eat half an apple. Even that slight change would deduct approximately 170 calories a day. The other 130 calories or so could be deducted elsewhere.

Of course, it's possible to defeat this kind of program by kidding yourself into believing that you ordinarily eat more than you really do. Let's say that you decide not to eat food such as the following on one particular day:

	Calories
One-half piece plain Danish	78
One-quarter cup bread pudding w/raisins	125
One brownie w/nuts	97
Total	300

These deductions are only going to be meaningful if, in fact, you do habitually and typically eat at least this many calorie-rich snack items every day. If, in reality, you typically have one Coke, one serving of ice cream and one brownie each day and then decide to go on having the Coke and ice cream while cutting out the brownie, it isn't going to help to imagine that you're giving up a Danish and the bread pudding.

Self-examination is not the only quality needed to know where to cut the fat out of your diet. Flexibility is also important. During the week, for instance, you may find that removing 300 calories more or less from your daily diet involves not much more than giving up one can of soda and a cupcake. On Sunday, though, it can be a different story.

	Calories
One-quarter cup stuffing	104
One-half tablespoon blue cheese dressing	40
One-quarter piece chocolate cake	90
One-half muffin	60
One-third pat butter	12
Total	306

As you might have guessed, this entire reduction was cut out of one meal—Sunday dinner. And certainly, these deductions can be made from a big dinner without forcing you to go away from the table feeling hungry. Yet they are perfectly valid as part of the program—*providing that you have typically been eating all these items or their equivalents every Sunday.*

Now that may give you the idea that you could go a bit further with calorie-cutting on Sunday than you can during the week. And that might very well be true—so long as you don't go *too* far. You might, for instance, have half a pancake less for breakfast and, later in the evening, substitute club soda for your usual alcoholic beverage. If you *are* able to do that, it is perfectly permissible to feel that the extra couple of hundred calories you cut on Sunday can be added back at some point during the week (a good time might be when you go out to a restaurant). Just be careful not to cut back *too much* on the weekends, because that could easily induce feelings of deprivation or even real hunger, either one of which could lead to a binge.

Another thing worth keeping in mind is that you should examine your diet very carefully for items that are relatively high in calories but don't give you very much satisfaction. It wouldn't make much sense to cut out half a corned beef sandwich, which has about 175 calories, when you could cut out two macaroons and eliminate 180 calories—unless those two macaroons are going to bring you more satisfaction than half a sandwich. And if brownies bring you untold delight, you're better off allowing yourself half a brownie on any given day than cutting out that special treat while leaving in four saltines, which have just as many calories as half a brownie.

Since it's possible that cutting out 300 calories every day could be a bit difficult for you to handle, especially while you're still adjusting to the new eating patterns you'll be learning, it might be worthwhile to take a quick look at what 200 calories can look like.

		Calories
One-half bagel w/cream cheese		110
One glass apricot nectar		107
	Total	217

		Calories
One-half cup mashed potatoes (made w/milk and butter)		99
One-half cup ice cream		127
	Total	226

		Calories
Seven french fries		149
One-half glass dessert wine		70
	Total	219

		Calories
Five potato chips		55
One doughnut		164
	Total	219

		Calories
One tablespoon jelly		54
Two chocolate chip cookies		102
One slice salami		45
	Total	201

Finally, we should point out that it's quite possible to lose all the weight you want to without ever counting calories at all. After reading this book and after paying more attention to your eating habits for a week or two, your consciousness of what you are eating will be raised to the point where you will probably be able to determine how much you are overeating, when and why, without recourse to any calorie charts. That knowledge will suggest ways in which overeating can be eliminated.

But even if it serves no other purpose, the calculations that we've done here will bring into sharp focus several important points:

- Removing too many calories from the daily diet is worse—much worse—than not removing quite as many as you would like to. Removing fewer than you would like will only slow down your weight loss; removing too many is very likely to lead to feelings of deprivation, which will in turn shake the foundations of your whole weight-loss program.
- A reasonable, realistic number of calories to cut out of the daily diet is 300. Many people will find that cutting out 200 or 250 is much easier to accomplish—which means that those people will get better results aiming for the lower daily deductions.
- It will not be difficult to find 300 calories that can be deducted from your daily diet without interfering with your nutritional needs or leading to hunger or feelings of deprivation. Snacks and second helpings should be your primary

targets, not main dishes. As you lose weight, you can gradually increase the deductions, because your requirements will be significantly less.

● In selecting foods to be eliminated, make maximum use of self-knowledge, experimentation and flexibility. Expect to have days that don't work out the way you had hoped; they will have no more effect on how long it takes you to reach your destination than hitting a red light does on a 100-mile drive. Just follow the map—you'll get there soon enough.

10

Use It and Lose It! Why Exercise Is Your Best Friend

There are many reasons why people gain weight, but if I had to give one reason that I thought was more important than any other, it would not be poor eating habits, the proliferation of snack foods or the disappearance of natural, high-fiber foods from our diet. If there is one overwhelming, single reason why overweight is such a problem, I would say it is lack of exercise.

And if I were asked to give one single life-style change that would be the most effective way to lose weight and keep it normalized, it would be to get more exercise.

Remember in the very first chapter how I listed eight common myths about weight control? I left one out. I thought if I included it, it would sound so entirely unbelievable as to make you think this book was written on a different planet. But now that you know I'm a down-to-earth kind of guy, here it is:

Most people who are overweight eat too darn much.　　T　　F

The correct answer is False.

Some people eat too much. But *most* people who are overweight don't.

That dismaying fact comes from several large population studies comparing the eating habits of normal and overweight people. And the majority of these studies concluded that overweight people—on average—eat no more than anyone else. In fact, they tend to eat *less*.

How can that be?

The answer to that question is the reason for this chapter. For most people, excess weight is the symptom of a deficiency of activity, not a surplus of food. Yes—overweight is most often a deficiency symptom. A deficiency of something just as important as vitamins.

For many, though, excess weight is most likely a result of too little activity *and* too much food. Especially fat-rich foods that turn into blubber a lot more easily than healthier fare.

Understand, it is entirely possible to lose all your extra weight without getting any more exercise than you do now, but you owe it to yourself to at least try to get more exercise, because it will make you lose weight *more quickly, easily,* and *healthfully.* Don't worry if you haven't gotten any exercise at all to speak of for the last 20 years. You can work into it slowly, and you can make it as vigorous or as easy as you like. In fact, if you haven't been getting any exercise, I'm going to *insist* that you make it easy on yourself, very easy, until your body adapts to your new habits. (If you're over 40 and have never exercised, it might be wise to check with your doctor—and possibly even have a cardiac stress test—before starting an exercise program.)

Why is exercise so important? The obvious answer is that it burns calories. That was the one benefit that everyone in our diet workshop named. A few people named a second reason: It makes you feel better. In reality, there are at least *nine* specific benefits that the weight-reducer can obtain from exercise, and each of them is tremendously important. The fact that so few people appreciate the *depth* of the benefits from exercise is probably one reason why so many simply choose to ignore it.

WHY EXERCISE IS ESSENTIAL

Before I tell you what these nine benefits are and how you can put them to work for you, let me take a few minutes to say something about exercise in general, because unless I do, you may think I'm exaggerating when I get down to specifics. What I want to say is that exercise is supremely important for one basic reason: It's *natural*. We human beings are physically put together with muscles capable of extraordinary exertion and with the capability of putting out work for hours on end. The people who made up the thousands of generations preceding ours made good use of these muscles and this stamina. When you consider the construction of the pyramids, the building of Rome and all the cathedrals of Europe, all of history's herdsmen, farmers, smithies and foot soldiers, and come right through the ages to our own grandparents and great-grandparents, who cracked coal and busted sod for 10 or 12 hours a day, six days a week, you can imagine that all the salt water in the world's oceans could well be humanity's collective sweat.

From the first day that man was created or evolved until the present day, our muscles have enabled us to do the work we *had* to do in order to survive. But in the course of all those hundreds of thousands, perhaps even millions, of years, *the relationship between our muscles and our bodies as a whole became one of mutual help and adaptation.* Because our muscles were used so frequently and so strenuously, we developed the ability to provide them with fuel by breaking down carbohydrates, fats or even protein. We developed efficient ways of providing this fuel on a short-term basis for quick bursts of energy and efficient ways of providing it for marathon feats of endurance. We developed ways of delivering larger amounts of blood to muscles when they need it and ways of cooling overheated muscles. We developed the ability to make our muscles grow larger and stronger if they were chronically being taxed past the point of their work limits. Our nervous systems developed the ability to program complicated movements into our muscles so that they could carry out difficult tasks without having to get fresh instructions from our conscious minds every instant.

But while all that was going on, there were parallel developments that have enormous consequences for people living in the age of automation. We adapted so well to strenuous, regular exercise that we actually came to *depend* on it. I mean that literally. *Now that we have learned to survive from day to day with very little physical work, the question is whether we can go on doing so very little physical work and survive from year to year.*

Ironically, lack of exercise is so common today that it's difficult to

point to any well-identified group of individuals and blame its problems on life-style. Only the extremes tend to stand out. We know, for
instance, that when a person is forced to remain in bed for several
weeks, debilitating weakness ensues, with loss of body protein, muscle wastage, loss of calcium from the bones and a greatly increased
danger of blood clots due to poor circulation. At the other end of the
spectrum, epidemiologists tell us that people who remain very active
into their later years will live to see *more* of those later years than their
sedentary counterparts.

But for most of us, the damage caused by lack of exercise is most
clearly seen when we reverse it with exercise. Some people have such
poor circulation in their limbs that they develop severe cramplike
pains upon walking a single block. When they are induced to do
therapeutic walking, going as far as they can until they must stop, then
resting, then walking again, their circulation increases and their
condition—intermittent claudication—often improves dramatically. People with varicose veins also benefit by walking, because the contrac-
tion of the muscles pushes the blood up through the veins and reduces
pressure inside those vessels. When people with serious low back
problems walk or do the right kind of stretching exercises, their
problem greatly improves and frequently goes away altogether, as
long as they continue their exercises. Arthritis often responds well to
swimming, yoga and other gentle forms of exercise.

Doctors who use walking or jogging as part of a rehabilitation
program for heart patients report that it lowers cholesterol, increases
high-density lipoproteins in the blood (believed to be protective against
heart attacks), improves or abolishes angina and lowers high blood
pressure. Exercise can lower a diabetic's need for supplemental insulin.
Psychiatrists are reporting that running greatly improves mood in
depressive patients, possibly due to changes in body chemistry. Other
doctors use exercise as a natural sedative for patients with sleeping
problems. Fewer complications have been reported at childbirth for
women who are allowed to walk around freely during the early stages
of labor. Migraine headaches are reported to be abolished by jogging
in some cases. Muscle tension and other symptoms of anxiety can be
made to disappear with exercise. There is some evidence that exercise
may be highly protective against gallstones, and animal experiments
as well as human studies even suggest that regular exercise can help
prevent cancer.

The fact that all these conditions respond well to exercise indicates how basic it is to our well-being. Robert Rodale, editor-in-chief of *Prevention* magazine, says that exercise is one of the best ways to continuously regenerate health and fitness.

So you see, although exercise may seem alien to you in your present sedentary life-style, your need for this wonderful friend is an important part of your heritage as a human being. And it's high time that you claimed that heritage!

LIGHT YOUR FIRE

Many of the more troublesome problems that we run across in life cannot be solved simply by direct personal action. There always seem to be complicating factors, like spouses, friends, enemies, money, conscience and time. Your eating problem is certainly one of the stickier sorts, but how encouraging, how motivating it is to realize that the mess created by that problem can literally be burned away, entirely on your own initiative and say-so! This is the first benefit of exercise. How wonderful if all chronic problems could be dealt with so directly and efficiently!

True, no matter how much exercise you get, you can't burn up your fat in a kind of bonfire; the process is more like applying the small flames of a craftsman's blowtorch. But that's actually good, not bad, because the more quickly weight goes off, the more quickly it comes back. And the more slowly it goes off, maybe, the more slowly it comes back. That may be even more true for weight lost through exercise than through dieting. In an important study of the effect of walking alone, in which women lost weight at the rate of about half a pound a week, Grant Gwinup, M.D., noted that "once a certain amount of exercise had produced a certain amount of weight loss, *that loss tended to be maintained with little tendency for a noticeable amount of weight to be regained.*"

The second important benefit or advantage of exercise is that *you do not have to eat less in order to lose weight.* It helps, of course, but it isn't a necessity. Those women mentioned before who lost weight through walking alone were told not to change their diets at all during the exercise period. In fact, most of them actually ate *more* than they did before, but they still lost weight. Although the calories burned by the most common forms of exercise do not seem exactly awesome, the cumulative effect over a period of months does—*even more awesome than the cumulative effect of overeating.*

To illustrate this, imagine that you've been gaining weight lately and put on about 6 pounds in the last year. By continuing to eat the way you have been, you could expect to put on half a pound in the next month. But suppose you began to walk an hour a day, *while continuing to eat just as you were before.* The effect of the walking would ordinarily be enough to cause you to lose about 3 pounds in a month, but even with the excessive eating you continue to do, you would *still* lose 2½ pounds.

I don't necessarily recommend exercising by itself as the best means to lose weight, because most of us find it isn't terribly difficult to cut a few hundred calories out of our daily diets without feeling deprived. But to the extent that reducing your food intake is difficult for you, exercise represents an easy way to reach your goal just the same. It's possible that the problem you have with your eating is of such psychological magnitude as to not respond very well to the principles in this book, or even the ministrations of a therapist. For you, especially, more exercise is the path of least resistance. And if you are substantially overweight, it's important to know that the heavier you are, the more calories you burn during any given unit of exercise. If you're a 200-pounder and spend an hour walking, you'll be burning up 350 calories, while your 125-pound friend walking along with you will only be burning 235 calories over the same time and distance.

Not having to eat less means that, besides not having to cope directly with your eating problem, you are also avoiding any possible problems that may arise from getting insufficient nutrition on a restricted diet. If you *are* changing your eating habits, as I hope you are, it means that you need only reduce your calorie intake by a very moderate amount to achieve good reducing results.

You may be thinking that for *you*, it would be easier to cut back on calories than to get more exercise, but don't give up yet. Don't even think about it! Later on, I'll give you some tips about how to get started with your exercise program, but right now, let's continue ticking off the benefits to be gained by becoming a more active person.

CHANGE YOUR MIND . . . AND YOUR BODY

The third benefit: Anything that makes you *feel* good is good for your reducing program. And nothing I know of makes you feel better longer, and deeper, than exercise. Whether it's a 45-minute stroll through the park, half an hour of jogging, a hike in the mountains or an hour of handball, exercise seems to make every neuron in your body purr with self-satisfaction. And the older you are, the better it feels. There is a warmth, a deep relaxation and letting-go that comes on you after exercise that makes you feel better all day and sleep better at night.

That's not poetry I'm spouting, but real fact. Blood tests show that prolonged exercise increases the production of certain substances that act as *natural antidepressants.* Other tests show that moderate but regular exercise reduces muscle tension. Ever wonder why you feel so good after an hour of square dancing or splashing around in the surf? It's not just psychological—rather, it's the classic interface of psychology and physiology.

It's nice to feel good all the time, but it's especially important when you're working on a major project—like losing weight. Anything that makes you feel jittery, anxious, uneasy, dissatisfied or depressed will make it that much harder for you to focus your attention on what you're doing. Exercise helps you make it easier on yourself.

Another good psychological posture during weight loss is to be actively engaged in a hobby. If you don't have one that's hot at the moment, a fourth benefit of exercise is that it can fill the bill very nicely. Taking up tennis gives you not only something to do but also something to think about when you aren't doing it. And not only does it fill your mind with images of yourself practicing the basic moves, but those images are of *an active you,* the best kind of you there is. A hobby like tennis or skiing or rock hounding also gives you equipment to buy, repair and worry about. Books to read. New people to meet. Trips to make. It gives your leisure time a definite sense of meaning, of momentum. It keeps you from getting into a situation where life consists of (*a*) working, and (*b*) avoiding the refrigerator.

If your exercise is walking around the neighborhood, that can be a hobby, too. I recently bought a softcover tree identification book, and I try to remember to stuff it into my pocket whenever I go for a ramble. I collect leaves and try to make more positive identifications when I return to my home. Another good idea would be to pay close attention to landscaping—assuming there is any in your neighborhood. If not, try to head for the nearest park. Parks were made for walking, after all, and as a taxpayer, why not get your money's worth?

Doing your own landscaping is also a perfect combination of

exercise and a hobby. Rock gardens, flower beds, stone walkways and fences all invite your loving attention and sweat. Vegetable gardens are a wonderful exercise hobby, too. And with gardening, you get the bonus of fresh, low-calorie, high-fiber food. Be sure to plant the rows far enough apart so that you can easily get in between them and weed. The right way to weed, by the way, if you're concerned about physical conditioning, is neither to bend over from the waist nor to squat. Rather, stand back a couple of feet from the weed and advance one foot so that the outside of your heel end is immediately adjacent to the doomed plant. Bend your knees and fall into a deep fencer's stance. *Keeping your back straight,* grasp the weed firmly with your gloved hand and yank it smartly out of the ground. Stand up, let your arm fly over your head and hurl the weed out of your garden. Find your next victim close to the row along the opposite foot and repeat, bending on your other leg. This exercise loosens up your hamstring muscles, strengthens the large thigh muscles and positively does wonders for your lower back. Throwing the weed away also keeps your shoulders loose. Each cycle, I'd estimate, is good for burning up 1 solid calorie. Maybe 2. The more weeds that grow in your garden, the more quickly you'll lose weight. That same lunging type of motion, done slowly, of course, is also a wonderful way to plant your seeds. If anyone asks you what you're growing in your garden next year, say slender.

The fifth benefit of exercise to the reducer is that when you lose a pound as a result of physical exertion, virtually all the weight you say good-bye to is nothing but fat. But when you lose the same pound through dieting alone, you are bidding farewell not only to some fat but also to anywhere from 2 to 10 ounces of lean tissue as well. A loss of lean tissue means you've lost part of those precious muscles in your legs that you count on to carry you around. The muscles that support your spine and hold in your stomach. Muscles you depend on for good posture and for holding your head up all day without getting tired. It may even mean a loss of connective tissue, cartilage and probably some of your bones as well. Have you ever gone on a crash diet and quickly lost 25 pounds or more? Did you feel tired, weak? Protein loss could be a factor.

In the studies I've seen, the amount of lean tissue lost by dieting alone ranges from about 10 percent to as high as 65 percent when the weight loss was produced by total fasting. With exercise, the loss of protein is minimal. In fact, with very vigorous exercise, you may well actually *gain* muscle mass even as you lose weight. When you combine a moderate reduction in calories, which we've suggested here, with exercise, the loss of lean tissue would be quite small, and perhaps nil, if you get enough exercise to create some new muscle tissue.

That new muscle, by the way, is going to give you two big bonuses. First, the pound of muscle you add by exercising is *more compact* than a pound of fat. I know several people who actually gained a few pounds with the diet-plus-exercise approach—but they looked and felt great. Certainly much slimmer. It seemed odd to them—until they learned that muscle simply doesn't make you look fat. But I also know more than a few people who have the reverse situation. They ask me why they look so chubby, when they actually weigh less than they did years ago. The answer? You already know it: Years of sedentary living caused them to lose muscle and replace most of the poundage with fat. That, plus the loss of muscle *tone* in the abdominal region, created the overall appearance of a person much heavier than mere poundage alone might suggest.

The second big advantage of more muscle and less fat is that muscle has a higher metabolic rate than fat. Even when you aren't exercising, your body needs to spend more calories keeping muscle tissue healthy than it does for fat. Result? More calories burned up, instead of piling up.

TORCH THAT FAT

During prolonged periods of starvation or strict dieting, the body is able to break down protein, play around with its molecules and come up with fuel that the muscles can burn. But ordinarily, it relies for fuel almost exclusively on carbohydrates first and fats second. And that second is a very distant second indeed. Chemically, carbohydrates are *ready* fuel, which can be quickly utilized for energy. Fat, even though it is a much more *concentrated* source of caloric energy, is mostly there as a backup system and has to be put through considerable engineering before it's ready to be socked into the muscles. If you run down the street to catch your dog, virtually all the energy you burn in that effort comes from glycogen, a carbohydrate stored in your muscles. The lard around your middle just lies there and watches.

But when you *really* get into exercise, taking long hikes or playing tennis or jogging, your body does some wonderful things. This is the sixth benefit of exercise. The body seems to realize that in order to pursue your new life-style, you are going to need a new system of fuel delivery. One thing it does is store more glycogen, that quick-burn fuel, right in your muscles where it will be needed. But much more important for our purposes, *regular, vigorous exercise increases your ability to burn fat, rather than carbohydrates, as fuel.* To put it just a bit more technically, your ability to mobilize and metabolize free fatty acids increases. Even better, this mobilization of fat as fuel in a well-trained person is a round-the-clock phenomenon: Experiments with animals reveal that it continues even under anesthesia!

Normally, the metabolism in "fat depots," as scientists call them (we call them bulges), is very sluggish. Increased metabolism in these areas may have something to do with the creation of bigger and better blood vessels in the area, which result from the body's need to send hot blood from exercising muscles up through the fat to the skin, where it can be cooled by exposure to air. In any event, it's clearly a beautiful example of adaptation, with your body changing itself to accommodate your changing needs. And the net result is that if you get into a regular program of vigorous, sweaty activity, those bulges, which may have seemed impervious even to your best dieting efforts, will begin to shrink noticeably.

The seventh advantage of exercise is that its benefits tend to be progressive. The exercise you do this week will make the exercise you do next week easier—encouraging you to do more. The first time I went jogging, as slowly as I could, I managed about 200 yards before I had to stop and get my breath. Three or four months later I had to run 2 or 3 miles just to feel as though I was warmed up. A year later, I ran 18 miles, up in the mountains, and *never* felt breathless, just more energetic. So you see, it doesn't matter how poor your ability or endurance is in the beginning. It's a wonderful experience to feel your stamina increasing week by week and to realize that you can burn away up to 600 calories an hour in the process of making yourself feel good all over.

Advantage number eight of exercise to the reducer is that group of health benefits we discussed earlier. I mean, I want you to live and to be healthy, so you can *enjoy* your new slenderness! As an overweight person, you see, you are particularly prone to a large number of health problems, and exercise can help abolish or prevent nearly every last one of them. That includes atherosclerosis (clogging of the arteries), high blood pressure, aches in your feet and legs, low back problems, poor endurance and shortness of breath. Overweight people in their mature years tend to develop diabetes, and exercise is now considered important in the treatment of this increasingly common disease, tending to lower the need for supplemental insulin. Statistically, fat people are even more prone to develop cancer, but at least one experimental study with mice showed that animals who were given vigorous daily exercise had much greater resistance to cancer than animals who did nothing but sit and dream about cheese all day.

COOL YOUR APPETITE

The final benefit of exercise—that I know of, anyway—is that when you get enough of it, the kind that makes you huff a lot and maybe even puff a little, it depresses your appetite. Yes, *depresses*. The common idea that exercising stimulates your appetite is completely false. It may be true for people who are underweight, but not for people like you and me. What's really happening, I think, is that as exercise normalizes a variety of your body functions, it also normalizes your appetite. It puts you more in touch with yourself, with your true needs, and removes you and your appetite from the grasp of mere habit. Possibly, this appetite-normalizing effect has something to do with a reduction in the circulating levels of insulin, since insulin is believed to stimulate the appetite. And fat people, remember, have abnormally high levels of insulin. It may also have something to do with the fact that the well-conditioned person is burning a greater percentage of fat, rather than carbohydrates, to provide energy. Since fat is such a concentrated source of energy, the body's master control may figure that there's no pressing need for large amounts of food and accordingly turn down the appetite a notch or two.

The fact that vigorous exercise normalizes appetite has not been convincingly demonstrated in a scientific way, but I know that it had that effect on me, and that many people who've seriously taken up exercise say the same thing. And one study with mice did show quite clearly that animals that were exercised in a rotating drum actually ate *less* than animals that were not exercised. My own feeling is that when a person who has become much more conscious of eating, as you have, takes up exercise, the probability that he will be able to eat less is very high.

NO-SWEAT EXERCISE

This past summer, I went to a wedding at the home of a woman whom I'll call Mrs. Garber. I hadn't seen her in about 20 years. The first thing I noticed was that she had seemingly gained a good 30 pounds, maybe 35 (strange, isn't it, how extraordinarily sensitive we are to changes of weight—in *other* people!). During the ensuing proceedings, Mrs. Garber certainly didn't stuff herself. In fact, she ate very lightly. Why, then, had she gained so much weight?

For all that we've said about the desirability of vigorous exercise, Mrs. Garber didn't get fat because she failed to take up cross-country skiing. In all likelihood, she became unhealthfully and unattractively overweight because *she stopped getting exercise that she didn't even know she was getting.*

Back in the days when we lived on the same street, Mrs. Garber, like everyone else, walked two blocks a day, just about *every* day, to get to and from the corner grocery store. It was common for women to go to a shopping area about five blocks away several times a week, and when they did so, it was almost always on foot. The drugstore that everyone went to was three or four blocks away, the dry-cleaning shop a block away, and the barber and beauty shop two blocks. And all of us walked. The row homes we lived in then all sat on a small embankment, and everyone had to walk up a dozen or more concrete steps to reach their front door. Inside each house, the bathroom and all the bedrooms were on the second floor, and the laundry was down in the cellar (we didn't call it a "basement" in those days). Each house had a garage in the rear, and after you parked your car, you had to walk up a steep flight of back steps to reach the rear entrance.

Today, Mrs. Garber lives in a ranch home. Everything is on one level, so she doesn't have to go up and down a flight of stairs every time she visits the bathroom. She doesn't have to go down the stairs and up the stairs carrying a basketful of clothing when she does her laundry. When she parks her car, she doesn't have to climb a steep set of stairs to get into her house; in fact, she may not even have to open her garage door, but simply press a button. Once in the garage, she gains immediate and direct entrance to her home. And, no doubt, she uses her car to do all her shopping nowadays. While she once had to lug packages back from the store and then up the steps, now she just puts them in the back of her car and that's that.

If you estimate the additional number of calories that Mrs. Garber was spending back in the old days, including all that walking and stair climbing, as well as having far fewer conveniences like automatic washer/dryers to use, you might come up with a figure of about 250 calories a day.

If people go on eating the same way they always have, but expend 250 calories less a day in physical activity, they will begin to gain weight and will continue to do so until they have put on about 25 pounds of flab. At that point, the caloric cost of carrying around the extra fat will stop the gain. The fact that Mrs. Garber looked as if she had gained more than 25 pounds may well have been a result of poor muscle tone in the abdominal region, which caused her belly to protrude. But the point is that it is extremely easy—almost logical, you might say—for someone to put on an extra 20 or 25 pounds simply as a result of moving from one place and one style of life to a more "modern" style of living.

Probably, if you are over 40 or 50, that true story about Mrs. Garber will sound very familiar. And so will her weight problem. Yet you may not have thought of your excess weight as being the result of lack of exercise, because you never considered walking to the grocery store or up and down a flight of stairs to visit the bathroom as "exercise." But it is. It may not give you the body of a Greek goddess, but it sure enough burns calories. And if failing to get that exercise inevitably puts pounds on, getting more of that kind of "invisible" exercise will inevitably take them off.

It would be convenient if we could get rid of some of our conveniences, wouldn't it? Jack up our houses 20 feet in the air so that we had to walk up the steps to reach the front door. And put the bathroom up on the roof. But we can't, any more than we can walk 3 miles down a suburban road with no sidewalk to reach the supermarket. So what we do is play games, weight-losing games that use spare moments here and there to bring back some semblance of an earlier and more active life-style.

Do you drive to work? Park your car a couple of blocks away and walk the rest of the way. Instantly, you are back to the days when you (or your parent) walked to the local grocery store. Want to speak to someone while you're at work? Instead of using the telephone, walk to their office. It's like walking down the street to drop in on a neighbor. Break time? Spend it walking; you just went to the neighborhood drugstore. Is there an elevator in your building? Use the stairs instead. Rest between flights if you want to, or even halfway up each flight if you have to. But *use* those stairs, just like all of us did years ago.

If you live in a house where there are stairs, consider yourself lucky. A staircase is the best piece of exercise equipment ever invented. Walk up and down every hour on the hour. Or every time there is a commercial break on TV. If you have more than one phone in the house, send the extra ones back to the phone company. Whenever you find yourself in front of the sink, do a half dozen knee bends (just go halfway down) and a half dozen toe-raises. Whenever you want to pick something up off the floor, use the same exercise we described for weeding. Talking on the telephone? Stand, don't sit, and do leg raises and semisquats. Use your imagination. Every little movement helps. If it makes you grunt, all the better. Here's your big chance to be a pig.

WALK AWAY FROM IT ALL

Changing a few little habits here and there is a good way to burn off maybe 50 to 100 calories a day. But in addition to that kind of exercise, you want to make vigorous, honest-to-goodness exercise part of your life-style. It will speed your weight loss, increase the mobilization of fat, make you feel better and help normalize your body chemistry. The best way for most people to do all that is to get into the habit of taking at least one long daily walk.

That's what I do now. When jogging produced a long series of injuries and a chronically sore back, I switched to walking. It was like heaven. All traces of back pain vanished. And I even lost more weight! Running was so stressful, I could only do it three times a week. But now I can walk five or six days a week, burning more calories. After a year or two, my enthusiasm was so great that I founded the *Prevention* Magazine Walking Club to encourage others to get the same benefits. Many thousands have joined, and their letters tell wonderful stories of weight loss and other health benefits.

Walking is something that requires no special training, coordination, skill or clothing. Well, it does require a good, comfortable pair of shoes, but that's about all. If you don't have such a pair of shoes, by all means buy one tomorrow. You can't pound nails with a hammer that is 3 inches long, and you can't walk with a pair of shoes that's too tight. Believe me, it will be the best investment you ever made, because walking *anywhere* is your path to salvation.

I've always thought there was something special about walking, ever since I read that Charles Dickens, my favorite novelist, used to spend practically all night walking the streets of London, mile after mile. Someone has said that the jogger is looking for something, while the walker has found it.

When I was younger I used to walk a lot because I had to. Now I walk because I have to again—not because I don't have a car but because I need the exercise. The town I live in, like many towns, has a hiking club, and that's how I got started. Many newspapers now carry schedules of weekend events, and chances are that a local hike is on the docket. Usually these hikes are easy, just enough to get you mildly sweaty, which is the best of all states to be in. But these weekend hikes should serve mainly to stimulate you and give you recreation. Walking once a week isn't nearly enough.

Earlier, I talked about getting started with walking when I was discussing how exercise can become a hobby. But the most important thing of all about walking is actually getting out there the very first time. It is that way with a lot of things in life. Taking the plunge is the hard part; the rest is easy. Objectively, it may not seem like there is anything very daring about simply going for a walk, but I'll be the first to admit that making a change in your daily routine is one of the most difficult things you can do. But it's also one of the most important.

The number of calories that you burn up walking depends on how much you weigh, your rate of speed and where you're walking. If you are toddling along at 2 miles per hour, which is about the speed at which you'd be going past an interesting showcase window, you will be burning about 145 calories an hour if you weigh about 120 pounds, 185 calories if you weigh 150, and 215 calories if you weigh 200 pounds. With moderate walking, at 3 miles an hour, you will burn between 235 and 350 calories per hour, depending on your weight. At 4 miles an hour, which is brisk walking, the kind you do when you're really serious about getting someplace, the values range between 270 and 400. If you are walking up a grade that is just steep enough to make you bend forward a little in order to balance yourself better, you will be burning up *twice* the number of calories that you would walking on the level. Don't, however, go out hunting hills the very first day. Work up to them slowly. If the weather seems uncomfortably cold for walking, be grateful, because walking in the cold air burns up 7 to 10 percent more calories than walking in balmy June weather—a result of increased metabolic needs to keep yourself warm and the burden of wearing winter clothing. Extremely hot weather also causes a small increase in caloric expenditure, but I don't recommend it. The best time to take your summer walks is early in the morning, while the sun is still low.

Be sure to keep a walking log and record your daily mileage. *Prevention* Magazine Walking Club members say the log they receive is perhaps their greatest motivational tool.

If you find your schedule somehow resistant to your best efforts to find time for walking, I want you to think about the following question, and give it a very serious answer: *What is the significance of the fact that you seem to have no time in your schedule to call your own?* To devote to your own precious health and recreation? Think about it. Is that a very wise life-style? Or even reasonable?

THE ONE BEST EXERCISE TO FLATTEN YOUR TUMMY

How can you tone up your belly without wreaking havoc on your back? Some abdominal strengthening exercises are anathema to those whose back muscles are also weak. While a fit individual can do straight-leg sit-ups until the cows come home, someone not so fit may find that maneuver nearly crippling. Instead, consider the Abdominal Curl.

Lying flat on the floor, keep your knees bent and your arms across your chest. Rise up slowly, curling up each vertebra separately until you're at a 45-degree angle. This means your lower back should still be on the floor. Lower yourself slowly, which is a complementary exercise called the Curl Down.

According to fitness authority Charles E. Kuntzleman, Ed.D., who calls this "the best exercise you can do," this simple movement uses only the abdominal muscles. Because you keep your lower back firmly on the floor at all times, you don't involve weak back muscles that could be injured.

(Be careful not to do this exercise with your arms behind your neck. The temptation is to pull on your neck, which could damage those muscles, warns Dr. Kuntzleman.)

Many women seem to feel that they'd somehow be "cheating" their husbands or their children by "selfishly" taking an hour of their time to devote to exercise. If that is your case, please take the time to think about another question: *Are you doing your husband or your children any kind of favor by wearing yourself out?* By not improving your health and appearance? Do you think they love you more because you spend every available minute at their service or in their company? Finally, ask yourself if it's possible, just possible, that by taking the time to exercise, to become fit, to become more slender, you might actually be improving your relationship with your family. No, it won't happen the first week, not usually. Men sometimes become childishly resentful and cranky when their wives begin to take time for themselves. Your kids may even laugh at you. But that won't last long, believe me.

Barbara worked on herself mentally for at least a month before she was able to get it all together and begin her walking program. Her husband greeted this effort with nothing but derisive laughter. Laughter gave way to mocking, and finally he even accused her of inviting the lustful stares of strange men. But Barbara persisted, never arguing with her husband or making counterremarks. Six weeks later, her husband suddenly announced *he* was going to begin walking, too. Now he enjoys it more than she does, and he never misses a day.

P.S. For information on joining, write to the *Prevention* Magazine Walking Club, 33 East Minor Street, Emmaus, PA 18098.

CHAPTER

11

Lose Weight and Add Years to Your Life!

If you are just a tad overweight, scientists throughout the world have been arguing about your fat for years. They have studied millions of people throughout their life spans to determine what that extra 10 or 15 pounds is doing to your health. The experts all agree that extreme obesity harms the health and shortens the life. But does mild or moderate overweight tax the body?

Yes, says JoAnn E. Manson, M.D., of the Harvard School of Public Health. Some previous studies on obesity and health have reached this conclusion; others have not. To set the record straight, Dr. Manson examined 25 of these studies. She found that each major study had at least one of three major biases, which led the investigator to underestimate the true impact of obesity.

WHERE DID THEY GO WRONG?

Many of these studies showed that the death rate is *highest* among the *thinnest* part of the population. That is why the Metropolitan Life Insurance Company—the folks who put together the standard ideal-weight charts that most physicians treat as gospel—revised the ideal weights upward by 5 to 15 percent in 1983.

But in one study, more than 80 percent of the thinnest men were smokers. "Cigarette smokers tend to be leaner than nonsmokers," says Dr. Manson. "That's probably because smoke boosts metabolic rate and interferes with calorie storage."

It wasn't being skinny that killed the men. It was cigarettes. "Failure to control for smoking's effects produces a misleadingly high mortality in lean subjects," says Dr. Manson. "Controlling for smoking means you have to compare overweight smokers with lean nonsmokers."

Other people slim down unintentionally when they develop a serious disease. In these cases, thinness is a harbinger, not a cause, of early death. So Dr. Manson recommends such people be eliminated from future studies.

To further complicate matters, several investigators, in trying to weed out extraneous factors such as smoking, got carried away and weeded out too much. They controlled for high blood pressure, diabetes and high blood-fat levels. That was misleading, since obesity boosts death rates by *causing* these three conditions.

HOW RISKY IS BODY FAT?

Once Dr. Manson fixed up these biases, she could finally get a clear look at how obesity can harm your health. And it wasn't a pretty picture.

"After controlling for smoking in the Framingham Study, the risk of death within 26 years increased by 2 percent for each pound of excess weight for ages 50 to 62 and by 1 percent per extra pound for ages 30 to 49," says Dr. Manson. "Which means that if somebody is 50 pounds overweight, he is 50 to 100 percent more likely to die in 26 years. He has close to twice the risk of dying as someone with an ideal weight. And he might lose 5 to 10 years of life.

"Even someone who's 10 pounds overweight has a slightly increased risk of dying sooner. And that person has at least a twofold to three-fold greater risk of getting high blood pressure and diabetes," she says.

WHAT'S YOUR HEALTHIEST WEIGHT?

So how will you know when you reach your healthiest weight? First run your weight by the old Metropolitan Life table (reproduced in Appendix A). "The 1959 table is probably more accurate than the 1983 one," says Dr. Manson. "It is less affected by the smoking bias, because the health effects of smoking were less apparent back then. The Metropolitan Life Insurance Company is now collecting data to release a new table."

Even if you weigh a little more than the table allows, you still may have a chance of being at your healthy weight. How do you tell? Take off your clothes and stand in front of your mirror.

Do you see rolls of fat or ripples of muscle? Is your frame petite and well padded or broad and lean? A table can't tell how much of your weight is fat and how much is muscle. So if you are unusually muscular or unusually large-framed, you can afford to exceed the average weight range without harming your health.

If you failed the muscle test, take a look at your fat. Where is it? "Where you store fat may be more important to life span than how much fat you have," says Dr. Manson. "Fat in the abdomen and the upper body is associated with high blood pressure, diabetes and blood fats more than fat in the hips, buttocks and lower body."

Now put your clothes back on. If you failed the test, have no fear. The good news is that if you reach your ideal weight, your body will forgive you! Your risk will return to nearly normal, studies show.

Of course, an obsession with thinness can be just as unhealthy as carrying around a big bundle of extra pounds. "Extreme thinness, as in anorexia and malnutrition, is unhealthy," says Dr. Manson. "And I know lots of people won't quit smoking because they're afraid they might gain weight. They should know that even if they gain a few pounds, they'll still be healthier if they don't smoke. A smoker of average weight has the same mortality risk as a nonsmoker who weighs 40 percent above average weight.

"I'm not advocating you eliminate all forms of fat on your body," adds Dr. Manson. "Everyone has a small amount of fat on the abdomen. And you don't need to be as skinny as those flat-stomached models in fashion magazines. It's just a matter of degree—a little love handle may be okay, but five are not."

PART

The
Weight-Loss
Guide to Food
and Nutrition

CHAPTER

12

How Natural Foods Can Help You Lose Weight

One of the most basic and healthful strategies you can apply in your weight-control program is to emphasize natural foods in your daily diet.

Notice I said "emphasize." I didn't say you have to (or even should) eat *only* natural foods. Nor did I say you have to eat unusual foods or shop only in health food stores. You can buy 80 to 90 percent of the natural foods you will need to hasten and help maintain your weight loss in any first-class supermarket.

Why should you emphasize natural foods? The answer to that one is easy: *Natural foods are much less fattening than processed or convenience foods.* There are exceptions, of course, but that's the general rule. Looking at it another way, natural foods are to be preferred because you can better satisfy your appetite by eating relatively larger amounts of them than you can by eating smaller amounts of high-calorie convenience foods.

What's more, we aren't talking about a marginal difference of 40 or 50 calories, but of 100, 200 or even more calories a day—and that's just from emphasizing natural foods, not eating them exclusively.

But just what *are* natural foods, anyway? That can be a mighty difficult and tricky question to answer if you try to frame your answer in highly technical or absolute terms.

To determine the relative degree to which a food is natural, all you have to do is ask yourself how close it is to the state in which it came from nature. The greater the number of additions, of subtractions and of modifications, the less natural it is.

And about nine times out of ten, these changes involve:

- The addition of sugar or other sweeteners.
- The addition of fats or oils.
- The removal of fiber.

Of course, there are other characteristic changes as well, most notably the loss of vitamins and minerals, the degradation of taste, the addition of preservatives, artificial coloring agents and other chemicals and the addition of salt (which can lead to retention of water and even high blood pressure). But purely from the perspective of weight control, the critical changes that occur in food processing are the addition of sugar, the addition of fat and the removal of fiber or natural bulk. The net results of these changes, needless to say, are unwanted and entirely unnecessary calories.

Let's get down to some specifics.

The potato is a perfect example of what can happen to a basically honest and nourishing food. Probably the most natural way you can prepare a potato is simply to bake it in its skin. Do that and you have something that is quite filling yet contains only 145 calories (less than two slices of white bread, and that's for a large potato). You get good vitamins, too, including 20 milligrams of vitamin C. As for fat, there's so little in a baked potato that analysis can discover only a trace.

Now if you were to eat french fries instead of a baked potato, you would probably eat about ten fries (each 4 inches long). But instead of getting 145 calories, you'd get 214—an increase of 47 percent, mostly from fat. And instead of getting 30 milligrams of vitamin C, you'd get only 16, a *decrease* of 47 percent.

Now let's say that instead of french fries, you were going to eat potato chips, but since they're taking the place of the french fries or the baked potato, you have to eat enough to satisfy your appetite. It's hard to say exactly how many potato chips that might be, but I'd estimate that if you were eating small chips, each only about 2 inches in diameter, you would wind up eating around 20 before you reached the same sensation of fullness or satisfaction you'd get from one baked potato.

But when you eat those 20 small chips, you're getting 228 calories, about 50 percent more than you get from the baked potato and a little more than from the french fries. (Again, the added calories come from fat.) And as for the vitamin C, you get only a miserable 6 milligrams.

LOOK OUT FOR "EXTRAS"

But that isn't the end of the story. Foods are not consumed in a vacuum, and we shouldn't look at them with the same narrow perspective that a scientist might use. Let's use the holistic approach. In this case, ask yourself what you're going to *drink* after you eat your potatoes. Eating a baked potato doesn't make you particularly thirsty, because 75 percent of it is actually water. French fries, however, are only 45 percent water, and potato chips just 2 percent water. Even more important, both french fries and potato chips are likely to be loaded with salt, which makes you thirsty. And when you're eating french fries or potato chips, what is it you feel like drinking to slake your thirst? Water? Not very likely. Chances are, you're going to drink soda or beer, adding empty calories from sugar to the empty calories from all the fat in the potato chips.

To be fair, we should probably assume that you're going to eat that baked potato with a pat of butter. But even with the butter, your total calories will be about 180; your total fat will be about half of that in the french fries and just one-quarter of the amount in the potato chips.

Fresh fruit versus canned fruit is another good example of the effect of food processing on calories. If you eat a peach for dessert, you get something sweet and tasty that has about 60 calories. If you eat a peach that was canned in heavy syrup, you get something that's *very* sweet, not all that tasty, and has 126 calories—a caloric increase of more than 100 percent. And that, mind you, is the smallest canned peach on the market. If you eat one of the largest kind, you get 170 calories!

Do you enjoy the taste of fresh blueberries? If you were to indulge yourself when they're in season by eating a whole cupful, you would be getting 90 calories. But eat the same cupful of blueberries canned and sweetened—a kind frequently sold in supermarkets—and instead of 90 calories, you're getting 229.

Do you like fresh sweet cherries? Eat a whole cup of fresh cherries and you've just taken in 82 calories—not all that bad for a delicious snack that's only available for a few weeks a year. But if you eat your cherries canned in syrup, that same cupful is going to sock you with almost 210 calories.

In fact, you'd be better off eating a whole cup of fresh cherries than eating just a half a cup of canned cherries—that's how many extra calories are added by the syrup.

If, instead of eating that cup of canned cherries, you were to have a small piece of cherry pie, the calories would climb all the way up to about 310. Choosing the pie instead of the cup of fresh cherries costs you 230 calories. At that price, don't you think you could learn to enjoy fresh, *natural* food as much as the cooked, sugar-laden pie? (To exercise away the difference between the two, you'd have to walk about 2 miles!)

With apple pie, it's the same story. One small piece of the pie has almost as many calories as four whole apples. Enjoy one good-size apple instead of a piece of pie and you've done as much for your waistline as you would by walking rapidly for three-quarters of an hour.

For breakfast, I often enjoy a whole grapefruit cut into wedges, which has about 80 calories. If, instead of the fresh fruit, I ate 1 cup of sweetened grapefruit sections from a can, I'd be slipping myself an *extra* 100 calories.

HOW FIBER FIGHTS FAT

Most of us probably know that foods with a lot of fiber take longer to eat and fill us up more. But how many, I wonder, realize that *including fibrous foods in your diet actually reduces the extent to which you can absorb calories from your food.* That most interesting fact was revealed in a study carried out jointly by the United States Department of Agriculture and the University of Maryland and reported in 1978. A dozen adult men were put on a low-fiber diet for 26 days and a high-fiber diet for another 26 days. Although their change in body weight, if any, was not reported, careful analysis revealed that on the high-fiber diet, there was a 4.8 percent decrease of calorie digestibility compared to the low-fiber diet. That's a significant percentage, amounting to 86 fewer calories a day absorbed on a diet consisting of 1,800 calories and 120 fewer calories a day absorbed from a diet of 2,500 calories.

Some people might object that this is not a fair comparison, because the low-fiber diet might have been unnatural. But I don't think it was all that unusual. A typical low-fiber breakfast consisted of grapefruit juice, puffed rice, milk, an egg, toast with butter and jelly, and coffee with cream and sugar. A typical lunch was a tuna fish sandwich with mayonnaise on white bread and a glass of apple juice. A typical dinner included vegetable juice, ground beef and macaroni, a white roll, grape juice and ice cream. Sounds pretty typical to me, although most people would have a piece of fresh fruit at least once in a while.

If the low-fiber diet wasn't all that different from what many people eat, neither was the high-fiber diet. In fact, I wouldn't even call it a "high-fiber" diet; it's just *relatively* higher. The only items in a day's worth of eating the high-fiber diet that did in fact include any fiber were grapefruit, puffed rice, a serving of dates, three pieces of white bread, a serving of corn, some pineapple tidbits, one serving each of spinach, carrots and cabbage, and blackberries.

In fact, the authors of the study—June L. Kelsay, Ph.D., and colleagues— purposely designed the high-fiber diet so it wouldn't include any whole grain products. Her idea, I suppose, was to see if a moderate amount of fruit and vegetables would make a difference in the excretion of calories and other nutrients. And, of course, it did. While 96.3 percent of the calories consumed in the low-fiber diet were absorbed, only 91.6 of those in the high-fiber diet actually passed through the intestinal tract and into the system where they could provide energy— and fat power.

It seems to me, although I have no data to prove it, that if you put some *real* fiber in your diet, you would get a substantially greater decrease in absorbed calories. And in fact, I suggest that you do just that. *Gradually.* Why go on eating white bread, when whole wheat bread not only tastes better but has so much more fiber? Do you *always* have to eat routine stuff like puffed rice or eggs for breakfast?

Why not try some hot oatmeal, with a teaspoon or two of bran mixed into it? Or some sugarless granola? As for lunch and dinner, I'd suggest that you make good friends with potatoes, beans, peas, soybeans, brown rice, carrots, cabbage and turnips. If you have any taste at all for slightly exotic grains, try millet, barley or buckwheat. You'll find plenty of excellent recipes for these kinds of foods in any good natural foods cookbook. Change your diet slowly, and don't continue eating anything you don't develop a taste for after eating it several times.

Focusing on these kinds of high-fiber foods will give you even more bonuses than a greater sensation of being filled and a reduction of calorie digestibility. High-fiber foods also tend to lower circulating levels of insulin, a hormone that is believed to stimulate appetite. They probably do that simply by making you *need* less insulin. One theory is that, with all that fiber, your food is digested much more slowly, and sugar is entering your system at a slow, steady pace instead of in one big burst. Another important bonus is that a high-fiber diet may tend to lower elevated blood pressure. In the study by Dr. Kelsay and her colleagues, 6 out of the 12 men had a diastolic blood pressure averaging 88 while they were on the low-fiber diet (80 is normal). On the high-fiber diet, the average diastolic blood pressure dropped to 78. That difference could be extremely significant, because diastolic blood pressure is not lowered all that readily.

Now, I don't want to exaggerate the importance of fiber to the weight reducer, because the truth is that fiber or bulk is not the only thing that signals your system that you're "full." Research indicates that the fat and protein content of the meal is also very important. In fact, it's perfectly possible to eat an enormous salad and still not really feel satisfied, because you haven't given your system any appreciable amount of protein or fat. Just the same, fiber is another factor in giving you that satisfied feeling. And it isn't just the fiber in natural foods that helps fill you up, but also their water content and crispness. Canned peaches, for instance, slip down the throat much more easily than raw peaches; eating three canned peach halves is no great challenge, but eating three raw peaches is.

Some foods that are usually thought of as natural really aren't all that natural (remember, natural is a relative word). In fact, two foods that have become the very symbols of "natural food" in the commercial marketplace have in truth been subjected to some "classic" food processing. I'm talking about granola and yogurt.

Granola.   Take a good close look at the ingredients label on some granola boxes—either in a supermarket or a health food store. The first ingredient listed may be oats, which means that there are more oats in the granola than any other single ingredient. But keep going. The second ingredient is probably brown sugar. Then, a few items down, you'll come to honey. What's happening here is that the manufacturer has divided the sweetening agent into two different sources in order to avoid having brown sugar as the largest single ingredient. Some manufacturers have three or four different sweeteners in their granolas: brown sugar, honey, corn sweetener, date sugar or dried dates and raisins can all be used to add sugar in one form or another (dried fruits like dates and raisins are loaded with natural sugars) without being forced by labeling laws to list sugar as the first ingredient.

Keep studying that granola label. Among the first few ingredients, you'll also probably find "vegetable oil," which might very well be coconut oil, one of the few vegetable oils containing saturated fat. What I really find objectionable about the oil added to granola is that many of the key ingredients in granola are already *naturally* rich in oil: all kinds of nuts and seeds, and even wheat.

The net result of these additions is a product that . . . well, just look at the label again. How many calories to the ounce? Probably somewhere between about 110 and 125. Some manufacturers list 1 ounce as "one serving," but while that may be true for a small child, in my experience the typical adult is going to eat at least 2 ounces at a time. Add another 80 calories for half a cup of milk and you're talking about 300 calories or so for a serving of granola. Not that there's anything wrong with a 300-calorie breakfast—but once more, go back to that label and see how much protein and vitamin value you're getting for those 300 calories. The answer will vary depending on the formula (some granola makers fortify their products with dried milk or yeast), but in general, between the cereal *and* the milk, you're lucky to get about 10 grams of protein (half of which comes from the milk, not the granola). For the same number of calories—about 300—you could have two scrambled eggs and a piece of lightly buttered whole wheat toast and get 17 grams of protein—70 percent more protein for your caloric money.

But what I personally find much more objectionable about commercial granola as a food for the weight-conscious person is that it can be eaten like candy right out of the box. And many people do just that.

In fact, it's even too easy to take a second and third helping of granola with milk. I can't remember ever eating a couple of eggs and a piece of toast and then going back and cooking a second helping, but I can remember all too well demolishing one-third or more of a box of granola at one sitting. And although I've experimented with making my own granola, using as little oil and honey as possible and fortifying it heavily with brewer's yeast, I find that I'm still unable to control my intake of this delicious "natural candy." So I've been forced to exclude it completely from my diet. If I want cereal in the morning, I have a bowl of hot oatmeal that I prepare with a lot of milk. I find it much more satisfying than the granola and I never even think about making a second bowlful.

I'm not suggesting that everyone has to exclude granola from the pantry, though. If you can control your intake, I'd suggest you prepare your own, going as easy as possible on oils, sugars and nuts, and fortifying it with dried skim milk, brewer's yeast and fresh fruit. Try to work some wheat germ and bran into the formula, too. But if you aren't going to make your own granola, think twice about having it around the house.

Yogurt. Just now I've gone to my refrigerator and taken out a familiar 8-ounce carton of yogurt. Looking at the label, I see that the contents have 150 calories. Do you have a carton of yogurt in your refrigerator? If you do, take a look at it and see what the calorie count is. If it's a flavored yogurt, like blueberry or strawberry, it probably has about 260 to 280 calories. Why the big difference? Simple. The kind of yogurt I've been eating lately is "plain." Don't be confused by the "low-fat" legend that most yogurts have. The important story about yogurt is not fat but sugar. Yes, plain, ordinary sugar. The small amount of fruit that's in a carton of flavored yogurt contains possibly 30 calories—which means that the rest of the extra calories—100 of the little buggers—are all from the sugar in the fruit syrup.

In other words, if you figure that a teaspoon of sugar has 15 calories (which we are assuming in this book, in keeping with the values given in government publications), your fruit-flavored yogurt contains the equivalent of 6 teaspoons of table sugar—and you say you thought yogurt was a *health* food?

Sure, yogurt is a health food—when it's really yogurt. When I traveled through the Caucasus region of the Soviet Union, I had yogurt, or a form of it they call *kefir,* almost everywhere I went. It's of a looser consistency than our yogurt and is served cold in a cup with a sprig of mint. You drink it down and it tastes pretty much like buttermilk. The calorie content of that kind of yogurt will vary with the fat content of the milk, but it will be somewhere between 115 and 160 calories per cup. If you make your own yogurt at home from whole milk, it will have about 160 calories—the same number of calories as are in a cup of milk. Commercial yogurt is often made from partially skimmed milk, often mixed with milk solids, so again, the calorie count can vary somewhat. But it probably won't go over about 160.

But even the "all-natural" yogurts that are flavored will typically have about 100 extra calories from the fruit syrup. As far as calories go, you might as well be eating a cup of yogurt into which you had mashed two-thirds of a chocolate candy bar!

Yes, you say, but . . . *plain* yogurt? It's tasteless!

Well, taste is a relative thing. Not so long ago, I felt the same way. But once I realized that fruit-flavored yogurt was loaded with sugar, I decided to give the plain variety an honest chance. At first I simply put in some chopped fruit, sometimes running it through the blender, and that added maybe 20 calories or so but also a lot of taste and a lot of vitamins A and C. Did it taste sweet, like commercial yogurt? No, I admit it didn't. But after a while, it began to taste *better* than commercial yogurt. After a few weeks, it got to the point where commercial yogurt tasted sickeningly sweet, like a child's confection.

And, believe it or not, in another few weeks I found that I was eating plain yogurt by itself and enjoying it. If that sounds a little difficult to believe, consider that to a person who's never drunk wine, a pale white wine tastes somewhere between dull and vaguely bitter. Sweet wines are almost always preferred at first, but eventually even the most occasional wine drinker learns to prefer the dry wine that he once thought was insipid. So you can *learn* to really enjoy plain yogurt, just as many people are learning to enjoy spring water instead of soda.

Actually, the way I enjoy yogurt most is to put about 4 ounces of the plain variety inside half a cantaloupe and add a heaping table-spoon of cottage cheese, which I blend with the yogurt. That whole delicious treat has a total of only about 185 to 200 calories, still significantly less than one carton of sweetened yogurt.

But yet—and this is an important point—the real purpose of eating natural yogurt with a fresh fruit instead of the sweetened commercial product is *not* simply to shave off calories. The real purpose, as I see it, is to eat a *reasonable* number of calories in the most totally satisfying form. In other words, if you typically make a lunch out of sweetened yogurt and one or two pieces of fruit, the total calories involved are not at all excessive for lunch. But by using plain yogurt and eating it with cantaloupe, you are getting something that is going to be more chewable, more filling and much more nutritious than the sweetened yogurt. For the person who makes a lunch out of sweetened yogurt and fruit, a good substitute for the apple and banana that might typically follow the yogurt would be a good, thick slice of homemade whole wheat bread or a somewhat smaller piece of a banana nut loaf bread made with whole wheat pastry flour and smaller amounts of soy flour. The calories from that lunch are going to be about the same as they were before, but the protein, fiber and mineral content will be considerably higher, and the whole affair will be a lot more interesting and satisfying.

IS MEAT A NATURAL FOOD?

What could be more natural than a juicy piece of meat? High in protein, B vitamins and iron, meat is one of the least processed foods we eat today. The one item that virtually all fast-food establishments feature is hamburgers, and if you go into an expensive restaurant you're likely to find the menu featuring the likes of steak *au poivre* and rack of lamb. At home, the family of modest means eats meat loaf while the wealthy family dines on strip steak. Italians are fond of veal, Germans of sausage and Greeks of lamb. Many of us are fond of all three, and a lot more besides.

Yet, there is something about meat—particularly beef—that many people regard as unnatural. If you go into a "natural foods" restaurant and ask for a steak, they'll look at you like you're mad. When the average person becomes interested in eating "health foods," one of the first things he's likely to do is cut down on beef consumption. People who are worried about their hearts do the same thing. Marathon runners, who are a long way from having cholesterol problems, often say they avoid eating red meat because it makes them feel sluggish. Vegetarians will say that eating meat is immoral or unnatural. Some consumers will admit that meat is a natural food, but because cattle are often fattened with the use of hormones, their meat is chemically tainted and should be avoided as unnatural.

But all that still doesn't answer the question of whether or not meat in general and beef in particular are basically natural foods. Neither does it address the role of meat in the reducer's diet.

To cut through the confusion around the subject of meat, we have to understand that there are basically two different kinds of meat: that which comes from wild animals and that which comes from domesticated animals. And the major difference between these two kinds of meat is the fat content.

The best examples of animals raised entirely in the natural state are marine creatures. Except for some pollution, the habitat, diet and life-style of ocean creatures probably hasn't changed since the days of Noah. But history aside, virtually all fish have an extremely low fat content. Sea bass and halibut, for instance, have just a little over 1 percent fat content. Shrimp and squid have a tad *less* than 1 percent fat, while the abalone is only 0.5 percent fat. Crabs and mussels are about 3 percent fat, and terrapins just a little bit more. Tuna and swordfish hit the 4 percent fat level, while mackerel is quite extraordinary with 12 percent fat content.

Freshwater fish aren't much fatter, on the average. Catfish are only 3 percent fat and carp 4 percent, while the lake trout is 10 percent fat. From this little survey, you can see that even when you lightly brush on some butter before baking your fish, the fat content isn't going to average very much more than about 5 percent.

In greasy contrast, the edible portion of the carcass of a choice-grade steer, the kind most frequently sold in supermarkets, contains 34 percent fat. The same meat from a prime-grade animal is no less than 39 percent fat!

The reason for this enormous difference is not simply a reflection of a difference in species. Rather, it is the direct result of the way these animals are bred and raised. And the most prevalent technique for raising livestock is to make them grow as quickly as possible and reach a certain level of fatness.

It's difficult to get accurate and truly comparable figures for the fat content of domesticated animals resembling steers, but some preliminary information I've seen from analyses done on wild antelope and zebras indicates that these animals have only about one-quarter to one-third the fat content of domesticated beef. Even reindeer, which are probably carrying some extra fat to protect them against cold weather, have a fat content of only 15 percent.

From this perspective, it's reasonable to say that the modern domesticated steer is an unnatural creature, in the sense that it probably couldn't survive in its present form if turned loose in the wild. If it *did* survive, it would be a lot leaner and tougher.

Chickens are usually considered to be less fatty than beef, and rightly so. A raw roasting chicken is only 18 percent fat, while a capon is 21 percent fat. There are no wild chickens flying around in the woods, but for the sake of comparison, the quail has a fat content of only 7 percent.

The rabbit is an animal that apparently has not been changed that much by breeding, so there isn't too dramatic a difference between the wild variety and the domesticated: 5 percent fat versus 8 percent fat.

To a weight reducer, the important thing about fat is that it is the most concentrated form of calories you could possibly eat.

Despite all that, I'm not going to suggest that you never eat meat again. Only that you eat it a little more thoughtfully.

While a good part of the extra fat content in beef is marbled throughout the flesh and is all but impossible to remove with a knife and a fork, many cuts of meat can be trimmed without difficulty. For every ounce of fat you cut away, you're saving yourself about 250 calories of blubber-power. By getting yourself into this one habit, you can eliminate anywhere from 500 to 1,500 calories a week, depending on how much meat you eat.

NATURAL FOODS CAN BE ABUSED

When some people go on a natural foods diet, they give up white bread, white sugar, soda, cake, candy and fatty cuts of meat. Instead, they eat lots of warm whole wheat bread covered with butter, honey dripped by the tablespoon into cups of herb tea, glass after glass of fruit juice, cashews, walnuts, almonds, dried apricots, prunes, dates, figs, raisins, unhomogenized peanut butter, sunflower and pumpkin seeds, fruit and nut loaves loaded with oil and honey, and even "high-protein" candy bars made with brown sugar instead of white. After a month of this, they get on the scale, discover they've gained 2 pounds, and can't understand why.

And I say that from personal experience. Because at one time, that's exactly what I was eating—everything except the candy bars. I was even eating ice cream made from goat's milk and sweetened with honey and carob, under the self-inflicted delusion that "natural" calories didn't count.

We already talked about how commercial granola and flavored yogurt are little better than snack foods. But you can get into big trouble with many others traditionally regarded as health foods. Because along with their high density of nutrients, many also deliver a very high density of calories.

Dried fruits, long popular as health food items, are perfect examples. Among other good things, they're unusually high in vitamin A and iron, two nutrients that tend to be scarce in many diets and are especially difficult to get in "finger food." Great. So you stock your refrigerator with prunes, figs, dates and dried apricots. And a couple of times every night, you raid your cache to get healthier and healthier.

But what some people seem to forget is that four prunes have 80 calories, four dates have 88 calories, four figs have 160 calories and half a cup of dried apricots has 170 calories. You may even develop a taste for dried, sweetened pineapple, good for 180 calories a slice.

Don't get me wrong. With the exception of dried, candied pineapple slices—which ought not to be sold in health food stores at all—dried fruits really *are* good food. You could even call them health foods and I would never argue with that designation. Only I'd call them dangerous health foods for people like you and me who have an eating problem.

Maybe what I'm saying is that we ought to redefine our idea of "health foods" to include fresh fruits of every kind as well as dried fruits. And that's certainly logical enough, since fresh fruit is more natural than dried fruit anyway.

With nuts, it's the same story. High in protein, B vitamins, iron, magnesium and trace elements, nuts are also, unfortunately, very high in oil. A handful of a dozen roasted almonds, which you can easily polish off in the time between the end of the late news and the beginning of the "Tonight Show," is a 100-calorie snack. A mere quarter-cup of dried pecan halves is also worth better than 100 calories. So are ten peanuts roasted in the shell (technically, peanuts aren't nuts—they're legumes, but who cares?).

Walnuts have a very warm look and interesting texture, so many people use them for interior decoration, keeping a wooden bowl full of them on an otherwise empty table. But if you sit down in front of that pile of edible decoration and take a nutcracker to ten of them, you've just ingested 264 calories. Which will not look nearly as pleasant on your thighs as they did on your table.

Again, don't get the idea that I'm against nuts. If you can eat them as food instead of as crunchy little things to keep your mouth occupied, you're getting excellent nutrition. But exercise the same cautions I described for dealing with dried fruits. Never sit down with a can or a bag of nuts in front of you. Don't leave nuts lying around the house, shelled or unshelled. Realize that nuts are food, like meat, and should be given the same respect. As a matter of fact, many excellent vegetarian recipes call for nuts because of their high protein, vitamin and mineral content. Incorporating them as an important part of a meal featuring grains or vegetables is probably the best way to enjoy the flavor and nutritional goodness of nuts.

There's no point, by the way, in buying "dry-roasted" nuts in hopes of saving calories. There's already so much oil *inside* nuts that the small amount usually used in roasting them makes only a negligible difference. What I would suggest, though, is that you buy unsalted nuts. Besides being more healthful, unsalted nuts (like almost any unsalted food) do not inflame the appetite the way the salty ones do.

Ditto for sunflower and pumpkin seeds. Great health foods. Brimming with protein and vitamins—bursting with calories. Half an ounce of sunflower seeds would fit very nicely in the palm of your hand: You're looking at 80 calories. Those are sunflower seeds that have already been hulled—the way nearly all of them are sold these days. But you can still get the unhulled variety in health food stores and I recommend those as a way of getting the good things that sunflower seeds have to offer without having to worry about eating too many too fast.

THE PROOF OF THE NATURAL PUDDING

While there are innumerable reasons why eating natural foods *ought* to help reduce your weight and keep you slender, proving it isn't all that easy. The one obstacle to carrying out a study that would prove or disprove my contention is that the majority of people who eat a diet emphasizing natural foods also get quite a bit of exercise, typically from activities associated with natural living: gardening, hiking, skiing, that sort of thing. They're also likely to be simply more conscious of their diet and their health in general. So it would be mighty difficult to find a group of people who are exactly like a "control group" in every respect except for their natural diet.

There is, however, a fascinating experiment we can look at to try to get an objective view of the relationship between natural foods and obesity. It was carried out by Michele Bremer, Ph.D., a nutritionist, and although published in abbreviated form in a nutrition journal, the complete study (actually done as her dissertation) has been published under the title of *An Examination of Some Aspects of Two American Diets* by the Soil and Health Foundation. What Dr. Bremer did was to feed a sizable number of test animals (mice and rats) two different diets, one composed of customary or "supermarket" foods and the other composed of only natural foods.

Half of the food used in the experiment was obtained from a well-known chain of restaurants that also manufactures frozen foods. That was called the "supermarket" diet. The other food was obtained from Fitness House, the then corporate kitchen of Rodale Press, which, as Dr. Bremer puts it, is "generally regarded as the center of the natural foods movement." Both groups of food were mixed into slurries, frozen and fed to the animals to eat as they wished.

Here are some of the typical items that were included in the "supermarket" diet: cornflakes and milk, chicken pie, chocolate pudding, meat loaf, milkshake, hamburger, apple pie, Cool Whip, french fries, spaghetti and meatballs, Jell-O, Oreo cookies, beef TV dinner, hot dogs and beans, bologna and cheese sandwich, filet of flounder, corn, vegetable soup and canned fruit cocktail.

Here are some of the typical items included in the natural foods diet: granola with milk, brown rice, chili con carne, polenta (a cornmeal dish), salad, cashew-millet casserole, fruit, cheesecake, corn bread, rice/wheat kasha, cherry crisp, peanut butter, liver with bacon and bananas with custard sauce.

After careful analysis of the contents, Dr. Bremer designed the diets in such a way that, although they contained different foods, *the calorie count, ounce for ounce, was almost exactly the same.*

For a period of months, which is a very long time in the life of a mouse, the animals ate their respective diets. When the appointed hour came, as it does for all laboratory animals, a representative sample was chosen to be autopsied and analyzed. A special effort was made to select from the supermarket group only those animals which appeared to be healthy. (It turned out that during the course of the experiment, the animals eating the supermarket diet, although kept in the same laboratory, developed skin infections which most of the "natural food" animals resisted.)

The analysis revealed two facts of major importance. First, the supermarket group was considerably heavier than the natural foods group. Perhaps even more important, they had a sharp increase in percentage of body fat, indicating that their increased weight was not in the form of muscle or bone.

Second, at one point in the experiment—which was actually a series of experiments—both groups of animals were given access either to natural foods or supermarket foods. Almost without exception, the animals chose the supermarket foods, probably because they were sweeter. That observation is important, because it shows that even animals may select foods which are unhealthful.

Dr. Bremer told me about another interesting observation, which was not included in her written report because it was not "scientific." She said that the man who was in charge of cleaning the animal cages told her that while the natural foods group permitted themselves to be handled during cleaning operations, the supermarket group was a very ill-tempered lot and exhibited frenzied and vicious behavior when their cages were being cleaned.

In another experiment, the same tests were repeated, using rats instead of mice. But in the rat group, the obesity difference for some reason was not found. However, the supermarket animals still had a higher percentage of body fat.

So make of it what you will. Are men more like mice or like rats? Or like neither? No real conclusion, I think, can be drawn from this study, but one finding that is at least highly suggestive is that in both instances, the animals eating what Dr. Bremer calls a "typical American diet" had a higher percentage of body fat than animals fed natural foods. And health scientists today are putting much greater emphasis on this fat-percentage measurement than on the more simplistic one of mere weight.

CHAPTER

13

Shopping Strategies to Make Your Thin Life Easier

Your behavior while marketing is critically important for two reasons.

First, it's difficult to eat food that you don't buy—unless you receive "care packages." Difficult, but not impossible, because in fact, most of us do from time to time get "care packages" from relatives and neighbors, usually cake or cookies. Then too, we may be eating 20 or 30 percent or even more of our daily diet outside the home. But still, for most people, home is where the food is.

The second reason that marketing is so important is that most people find it much easier to select their food wisely when it's sitting on a shelf or in the store freezer than when it's in their own refrigerator or in a bowl on the dining room table.

But that doesn't mean it's easy to get out of the supermarket carrying only the foods that in your most conscious moments you would choose to ingest and have become a part of your body. In fact, it becomes more and more difficult each year: The supermarkets go to great pains to take care of that. And too often, we play right into their hands.

In your typical supermarket, for instance, you will probably find more different kinds of soda than you will fresh fruits and vegetables put together. You might easily find 30 or 40 different kinds of cookies and 20 different kinds of crackers; if you can find one kind of whole wheat flour, you're lucky. If you have to go to a section of your supermarket that carries infant needs, you'll probably be forced to pass a gigantic candy and snack food section. In the supermarket closest to my house, you can't go to the area where such staples as eggs and butter are sold without passing a huge bakery section and rack after rack of pretzels, potato chips and corn chips.

In that same market, the shopper looking to buy some frozen vegetables will be forced to take in a long eyeful of every imaginable kind of frozen cake and pie, all of them beckoning, "Buy me!" with gorgeous color photographs.

Supermarkets, of course, do everything possible to try to encourage such impulse buying. Junk food is often placed in the immediate vicinity of staples. Large end-of-aisle displays most typically feature soda, cookies, crackers, marshmallows, etc. Walk down the aisle where fruit is sold and you may find that every 15 feet there is a big jumbled display of candy. That's a double trap: They're selling you candy when you're shopping for fruit or vegetables, and cashing in on the fact that people are more likely to buy candy when it's offered in a big jumble, as opposed to when it's neatly stacked on the shelf. Now that I think of it, it's a triple trap, because the goodies on display are exactly at eye level with a 5- or 6-year-old child.

But you aren't even safe when you're in the checkout line, because there you're apt to find more eye-level displays where cranky kids can reach out and ease their boredom with candy bars. Adults, too, are apt to be tired and hungry by the time they reach the checkout counter and are not above munching on a candy bar to soothe themselves.

Even in "health food" stores, you're likely to find the area around the cash register covered with all kinds of candy bars and confections. The fact that they're made with honey or brown sugar instead of white sugar is no saving grace to the person with a weight problem. At the health food store where I often do some shopping, the candy bars are on one side of the cash register, and on the other side are gallons of ice cream and jars of fresh-ground peanut butter.

GIRDING YOUR LOINS

At our workshop sessions, everyone agreed it's poor strategy to go shopping when you haven't eaten for several hours or more. Shopping when you're hungry only adds the force of true biological hunger to all the hidden and not-so-hidden persuaders that the supermarket has engineered to sell you "fun" foods that you had no intention of purchasing. Fighting off biology *and* psychology at the same time is no easy trick!

Yet three out of four of our workshop participants admitted that they *did* shop when they were hungry—usually right after work. This is a classic example of how the force of habit—sheer habit—pushes you toward overweight even when you realize full well what's going on.

Equally as unwise, and maybe even more so, is shopping on Saturday afternoon after you've spent all morning running around from one store to another. You're hungry, your blood sugar is low, and you're so fatigued that you're almost dizzy. Shopping in that condition not only lowers your resistance to junk food but might even give you the idea that you *deserve* some nice, rich goo as a reward for having run yourself ragged. Somehow it never occurs to us that what we're really saying is, "I've been working so hard that I deserve to get just a little bit fatter."

Resolve right now that if you do fall into any of the patterns we've described, from here on in you're going to shop only after you've eaten a solid meal. My guess is that the best time of all is early in the day, so consider doing your marketing after eating a hearty breakfast on Saturday morning.

By now it has probably occurred to you that it would be a good idea to take a shopping list into the market and buy only what you've decided—in your most rational mind—that you really want. I agree that lists are a good idea, and I urge you to try making a list for at least a few weeks. You may find that it will not only help you avoid unwanted snack items but also encourage you to buy more of what you would truly like to be eating—items like fresh fruit and vegetables, salad greens, cottage cheese and fish.

Another benefit of shopping with a list is that you can buy all the ingredients you need to make new recipes. And making new recipes is a fine idea for anyone trying to improve his eating behavior. For one thing, it's a positive, pleasantly challenging way to break out of habitual eating patterns (like spaghetti and meatballs and garlic bread dripping with butter every Wednesday night). Creating new dishes also makes you more sensitive to the taste, texture and aroma of food, which—although it may be surprising—is actually a good way to help gain control of your eating. That's because a great bulk of our overeating is done not with strange or new foods but with the most familiar items—french fries, chocolate chip ice cream, pretzels and so forth. But not having one or two key ingredients, I've found, is a common barrier to creating exciting new dishes. That's where your food list (and a couple of good cookbooks) can save the day.

The last thing I want to say about lists is that you should have one or two snack items on yours, to keep the list realistic and to remind yourself that you aren't *depriving* yourself of all snacks. And think for a while before deciding what snacks you want on that list. They should be foods that have a very enjoyable taste and that—if possible—leave you with a satisfied feeling. Pretzels would be a good example of a snack that will appear on very few lists indeed. Have you ever said—or heard anyone else say—"Wow, what delicious pretzels!"? They aren't very satisfying, either. In fact, because they're so salty, they also encourage you to drink soda or beer. The same goes for potato chips. On the other hand, if you really love brownies, decide ahead of time that you are going to buy two or three and really enjoy one with a glass of milk or a cup of coffee twice a week.

It's quite possible that after a month or two of your new eating behavior, you may not really want any snacks other than something like hard, juicy apples when they're in season or a plump honeydew melon. But if you've been accustomed to eating quite a few snacks, you'll probably find that your new program will be more successful if you don't give up all your snacks "cold turkey."

Having said that, you should select the snacks you enjoy the very most, and despite the fact that the Prevention System of Natural Weight Control does not tell you what to eat and what not to eat, I'm nevertheless going to list a group of snack items that I think you ought to at least *consider* never buying at all. They are:

- Candy
- Chocolate chip cookies
- Corn chips
- Fig cookies

- Macaroons
- Marshmallow cookies
- Peanut-butter-and-cheese-cracker "sandwiches"
- Potato chips
- Pretzels
- Soda

What makes these particular snack items so unwelcome? Several things. First, they are little hand grenades of calories, with one lumpy macaroon packed with 90 of them and one chocolate chip cookie with 51. Second, there is something about these items that makes it difficult to quit eating them once you have started. Third, with the exception of the fig bars, they are junk food, impure and simple.

YOUR PERSONAL DANGER FOODS

There are probably other items you shouldn't buy at all, but only *you* know which they are. They are the foods that you simply can't resist, the ones you either gorge on or nibble constantly. Take peanuts, for example. Theoretically, they are a fine food for almost anyone: high in protein, unprocessed, free of sugar and good tasting, they also come naturally in small sizes and keep a long time without spoiling, so that it's easy to just eat a few. Alas, all that is only true *theoretically*. For me at least, a bag or a can of peanuts is nothing but a fat-producing machine. Because I *can't* eat just a few of them. For years, whenever they were in the house, I would grab them at about 10:00 or 11:00 P.M. and eat them until my stomach almost ached. For the last year, peanuts have been on my *never* list.

Because I have very little self-control when it comes to food that is sitting in front of me, there are *lots* of items that I reject right at the supermarket, where, luckily, the temptation to buy them is only about 1 percent as strong as the temptation to eat them when they're on the kitchen counter or in the refrigerator. These items include just about all kinds of dried fruits—apples, pears apricots, figs, dates, even raisins—except prunes, which for some reason I am able to eat with some semblance of rationality.

Just as you will have to decide what foods to exclude completely from your shopping list, you can also choose the snack foods that you bring home for yourself or for your family partly on the basis of your ability to control yourself when eating them. If you know, for instance, that you can sit down and eat three or four walnuts and be done with them, then walnuts might be a fine, nutritious snack for you. If your family loves strudel, and you can enjoy and be satisfied with a 2-inch slice a couple of times a week, then there's no reason why you shouldn't buy strudel. At the same time, reflection may reveal that something that many other people find quite innocuous—like English muffins, for example—are for you an irresistible snack.

Self-inquiry like the above can also be applied to food items that are not usually thought of as snacks. For some people, cold cuts and delicatessen items like sliced ham or potato salad are strictly "meal" foods. But reflection may reveal that for you, they are not only meal foods but compulsive snacking items, too. Do you get an irresistible urge to make a salami and cheese sandwich at 11:00 P.M. when you know those foods are in the refrigerator? Is a 400-calorie wallop like that a reasonable part of your daily diet? Think about those questions and then decide if perhaps you would be better off not buying them at all.

I picked delicatessen items to illustrate this principle for a good reason: In general, foods sold in that section of your supermarket are high in price, high in preservatives, high in salt and high in fat. They also perish quickly—which encourages you to eat them quickly.

For many people, the greatest challenge in shopping is posed by the fact that they are shopping not only for themselves but also for the rest of their family. What do you do when other family members (who may or may not have eating-behavior problems) expect you to bring home cupcakes, ice cream, potato chips and other snacks you have a weakness for?

Many people will find that situation a convenient excuse to bring home junk food, telling themselves that it's for someone else when they know perfectly well that *they* are going to overeat the snacks. And I don't say that self-righteously, either, because I used to do it all the time. I'd buy Fig Newtons and tell myself that they were relatively healthful snacks for the kids because of the figs, never admitting that I ate twice as many of them as the kids did. It was the same with ice cream, only more blatant: I used to "buy it for them," but somehow I always managed to select flavors I liked and they didn't!

So the first thing to do is to sit down and objectively decide if you're playing your own version of this very juvenile and very fattening game.

If you are, that's great, because your course of action is clear: Buy snacks *they* like and you don't. If they want cakes and pastries, get some that have fillings that are acceptable to them but not at all appetizing to you. Get flavors of ice cream that bore you or turn you off but that others can enjoy.

CHAPTER

14

Be Alert for These Dieters' Deficiencies

Bad nutrition can produce bad health.

Hospitals learned that lesson, says Peter Lindner, M.D., director of continuing medical education for the American Society of Bariatric Physicians (obesity specialists). "That's one of the reasons they added nutritional support services," says Dr. Lindner, who also heads the Lindner Clinic in suburban Los Angeles. "They discovered that some common postoperative infections were not due to the surgery but to poor nutrition."

Researchers have found that immune-system response drops in people on very low-calorie diets, says Dr. Lindner. "In one study, the researchers were interested in the changes in disease-fighting white blood cells when exposed to vaccine. What they found was that the immune response was reduced in those individuals on improperly administered ultra-low-calorie diets, making them more subject to infection. That is probably one of the most dangerous aspects of very low-calorie diets."

If you're a dieter—and surveys show two out of three are—there's a very good chance you may be endangering your health, warns Dr. Lindner. You may be able to take nutrition for granted when you're eating like a horse, but it becomes critical when you start eating like a bird.

"A good balanced diet in the higher caloric range probably gives you all the vitamins and minerals you need. It gives you some leeway to play with," says Dr. Lindner. "Drop it down to 800 or 1,000 calories and everything counts."

In fact, according to the Food and Nutrition Board of the National Academy of Sciences—which sets our Recommended Dietary Allowances (RDAs)—it is difficult to get adequate nutrition on diets that provide less than 1,800 to 2,000 calories. Most popular reducing diets call for 1,200 or less.

A NUTRITIONAL BALANCING ACT

It's hard enough to juggle the four food groups into a nutritionally balanced diet when you've got a few thousand calories to work with. Dieters have a tougher task. They have to concoct three healthful meals with roughly half the calories they're used to consuming. And they start out with a handicap—they don't know beans about nutrition.

Following a diet guide may not help. Many popular diet plans are full of dubious nutritional advice. Most dieters know only enough to plan a 1,200-calorie menu down to the last morsel. But knowing calories isn't enough. You can create three low-calorie meals a day without ever straying from the candy counter.

Perhaps the most important thing to remember when you're counting calories is that it's the nutritional value of the calorie that counts. If you don't know the value of a calorie, you don't know what you're missing.

But Paul Lachance, Ph.D., does. Dr. Lachance, professor of nutrition and food science at Rutgers University, evaluated the nutritional content of 11 published weight-loss diets. He chose the 11 because they ran the gamut of popular weight-reducing plans—from high-protein/low-carbohydrate to low-protein/high-carbohydrate, with variations in between. They carried such familiar names as Scarsdale, Stillman, Atkins and the Beverly Hills Diet.

Using the RDAs as a frame of reference, Dr. Lachance and associate dietitian Michele C. Fisher, Ph.D., found that most of the diets were low in thiamine, vitamins B_6 and B_{12}, calcium, iron, zinc and magnesium. Thiamine, vitamins B_6 and B_{12} and magnesium were often at levels of less than 70 percent of the RDA. One diet, the Beverly Hills Diet, supplied less than 70 percent of the RDAs for more than half of the vitamins and minerals evaluated, and was so low in protein that researchers predicted it would lead to a serious protein deficiency over a long period of time.

And there's the rub. Most diets are protracted, if not forever. "Most people stay on a diet for a long time. After all, weight loss doesn't occur overnight," says Dr. Lachance. "If a diet lasts only two weeks, the vitamin and mineral loss is not going to be significant. As far as I'm concerned, women are dieting all the time and may have other risk factors—smoking, contraceptive-pill use—that can affect nutrient metabolism. For them, the loss can be very significant."

In fact, researchers studying otherwise healthy men found that even without those extra risk factors, a prolonged low-calorie diet had a damaging effect on their health. One group, which had previously eaten over 3,000 calories daily, ate about half that for a period of six months. Even though they were eating more calories than prescribed by most reducing diets, the men suffered from depression, anemia, edema, slowing of heartbeat and loss of sex drive. They also tired easily and lacked endurance.

Some weight-loss regimens, specifically those that are mainly protein, can lead to a potentially serious condition called acidosis, which also can occur on fasting diets. In one study, people fed a diet of solely protein and fat lost about 2 pounds a day—along with large amounts of nitrogen and salt in their urine. They suffered from the symptoms of acidosis, which can include weakness, malaise, headache and heart arrhythmias.

Acidosis can be remedied by adding as little as about 3 ounces of carbohydrate to the diet.

Needless to say, bizarre diets that rely heavily on one food—such as grapefruit—are going to be nutritionally bankrupt. Very low-calorie liquid diets can be deadly.

SPECIAL ADVICE FOR WOMEN

Women are always going to have to pay extra attention to the nutrient content of their diets because of their increased needs for certain nutrients. "For women, it's hard enough to get things like calcium and iron," says Cindy Rubin, clinical nutritionist with the obesity research group at the University of Pennsylvania.

Women generally need more iron and calcium than men. "Many women are going to have to supplement their diets with calcium and iron," says noted weight and fitness expert Gabe Mirkin, M.D., who ordinarily doesn't advocate dietary supplements. "One out of four women between 12 and 50 is iron deficient."

Though an iron deficiency may eventually lead to anemia, it has its own immediate health consequences. "When you're iron deficient, even though you're not anemic," says Dr. Mirkin, "you can't clear lactic acid as rapidly as normal from your bloodstream, so you tire earlier at work and play."

"The problem with calcium is that it's scarce except in milk products—the first thing many dieters cut out. Unless you choose skim milk, dairy products can be high in fat and calories," says Dr. Lindner. "It's difficult to get adequate calcium without milk unless you want to eat sardines, small bones and all."

How food is prepared may also affect a dieter's nutrition. "If you're eating a salad that was tossed three days ago, vitamins are lost simply by exposure," says Dr. Lindner. "If food is cooked too much, you can lose more. Especially at risk are the water-soluble vitamins, such as C and B vitamins."

One of those B vitamins is folate. Women are particularly at risk of developing anemia when they aren't taking in enough folate, which is found in leafy greens. A form of anemia occurs when there isn't enough folate in the body to produce red blood cells. Folate deficiency also has been pinpointed as a factor in a precancerous condition called cervical dysplasia.

Studies have also shown that low-calorie and starvation diets can lead to an excessive loss of zinc, possibly as a result of tissue breakdown. Researchers at the Veterans Administration Hospital in Hines, Illinois, found that weight-loss diets between 600 and 1,240 calories can be zinc deficient, depending on the type and source of dietary protein from which the zinc is derived. Diets that derive most of their protein from red meat tend to supply more zinc than those that rely on chicken, fish, milk products and eggs, which are, unfortunately, the main protein sources of many low-calorie diets.

If it all sounds discouraging, rest assured that the obesity experts understand—and have more than one solution to a dieter's nutritional dilemma.

- If you don't feel you can add red meat to your diet, or if time and money constraints make it impossible to eat only freshly prepared foods, you can take supplements. "Theoretically, it's not necessary to supplement your diet," says Dr. Lindner, "but realistically most people don't have the knowledge or the time to do it right. Especially if you're a woman, a standard multiple vitamin that contains iron, B_6, folacin [folate] and zinc, along with a calcium supplement, should help you make sure you're getting all of the 26 micronutrients you need."
- Learn the value of a calorie. You know there's a big nutritional difference between a 200-calorie candy bar and a 200-calorie protein salad. But even so-called diet foods aren't created equal. "Choose nutrient-dense foods," suggests Cindy Rubin. "For instance, eat broccoli as opposed to lettuce. Both are low in calories, but lettuce is mainly water. You're not getting the heavy doses of vitamin A you get in broccoli."
- Go for variety. Not only is it the spice of life, but it improves your chances of getting all the vitamins and minerals you need.
- Plan your diet menu from the four basic food groups. "Each of the major categories represents certain vitamins and minerals," says Dr. Mirkin. "Grains and cereals, for example, give you E and the B vitamins. Fruits and vegetables supply C and A. If you take in at least 1,500 calories a day and distribute your calories over the four food groups, you'll probably be taking in the nutrients you need."

EAT MORE AND LOSE?

The final piece of advice is something of a blockbuster: Eat more calories. By eating more, naturally, you're more likely to meet your nutritional needs. But will you lose weight? Yes, say the experts, as long as you burn up some of those calories through exercise.

In his book *Getting Thin,* Dr. Mirkin advises eating 1,500 calories a day—and using an hour of exercise to burn off 300.

The Weight-Loss Guide to Food and Nutrition

There are some unique advantages to this plan. Aside from losing weight healthfully, you'll stimulate your metabolism to burn even more calories. "You see, diets don't work," says Dr. Mirkin. "When you go on a diet, your metabolism slows down. When you're lying in bed, not even moving, you burn 60 calories an hour. If you're on a diet, you burn only 50. If you exercise, you burn 70—without even moving. Exercise speeds up your metabolism 24 hours a day, not to mention suppressing your appetite."

Dr. Mirkin recommends picking two sports—aerobic dancing and biking, for instance—and working up slowly to an hour of each on alternating days. "I specify two sports because it takes you 48 hours to recover, so you should rotate the stressors on your body," he says.

Older people especially need exercise as an integral part of any diet plan. "The two have to be together," says Dr. Lachance. "When you're young, your metabolism is higher and you can get away with more. When you get older, your body changes. Your metabolism slows, your lean body mass goes down and your propensity for adipose [fat] tissue goes up. You lower your need for calories, so if you don't add exercise, you get fat."

CHAPTER

15

Drink Up and Slim Down

Which has more calories: a nut-filled brownie or an accompanying glass of milk; a mug of beer or a whiskey sour; a glass of orange juice or a glass of Coca-Cola?

If you don't have a clue, it's probably because you're not used to thinking about the calorie content of beverages. After all, solid food is where most of the world's calories lurk, right? Serious weight watchers fret about the fattening possibilities of gingerbread cakes, pumpkin pies and oversized eclairs. But who cares about liquid calories?

Maybe we all should. For some people, beverages may account for close to 50 percent of total calorie intake. For most of us, the percentage is probably far higher than we think. And there are scores of drinks with higher calorie counts than any of the above sinfully caloric desserts. Besides, it's easier to substitute a low-calorie beverage for a high-calorie one if you know where all the calories are hiding.

Lesson number one: A glass of whole milk packs 159 calories but a brownie only 97; a mug of regular beer has about 150 calories but a whiskey sour, 184; and a glass of Coke carries 144 calories but a glass of orange juice, 112.

You'll find more surprises here. Our information comes from government nutrition data banks, manufacturers and, in some cases, from laboratory analyses.

Here's to a wiser and slimmer you!

BEVERAGE CALORIC GUIDE

Beverage	Serving Size (fl. oz.)	Calories per Serving (approximate)	Calories per Ounce (approximate)
Fruit Juices			
Apple cider	8	118	15
Apple juice	8	118	15
Knudsen cherry cider	8	96	12
Apricot nectar	7	125	18
Guava nectar	6	300	50
Pear nectar	5½	100	18
Knudsen papaya nectar	8	104	13
Libby's peach nectar	6	90	15
Cranapple juice, low-calorie	8	43	5
Cranapple juice, regular	8	173	22
Cranberry juice cocktail, low-calorie	8	48	6
Cranberry juice cocktail, regular	8	141	18
Crangrape juice	8	144	18
Cranprune juice	8	154	19
Grape juice	8	170	21
Prune juice	4	92	23
Grapefruit juice, canned	8	101	13

Drink Up and Slim Down

Beverage	Serving Size (fl. oz.)	Calories per Serving (approximate)	Calories per Ounce (approximate)
Grapefruit juice, fresh	8	96	12
Knudsen pink grapefruit juice	8	76	10
Limeade, from frozen concentrate	8	100	13
Lime juice, from concentrate	1	4	4
Lemon juice	1	6	6
Orange juice, canned, unsweetened	8	120	15
Orange juice, fresh	8	112	14
Orange juice, frozen, reconstituted	8	122	15
Orange juice, imitation (Awake, Bright and Early, etc.)	8	120	15
Tangerine juice	8	122	15
Five Alive juice	8	114	14
Pineapple juice, canned, unsweetened	8	138	17
Acerola juice	8	56	7
Coconut milk (liquid from mixture of coconut meat and coconut water)	8	605	76
Coconut water (liquid from coconuts)	8	53	7
Blackberry juice, canned, unsweetened	8	91	11
Tangelo juice	8	101	13
Winter Hill apple-apricot juice	6	95	16

(continued)

BEVERAGE CALORIC GUIDE—*Continued*

Beverage	Serving Size (fl. oz.)	Calories per Serving (approximate)	Calories per Ounce (approximate)
Fruit Juices—*continued*			
Winter Hill apple-raspberry juice	6	88	15
Winter Hill apple-strawberry juice	6	88	15
Mott's apple-grape juice	8	113	14
Pineapple-orange juice	8	126	16
Pear-apple cider	8	100	13
Pear-grape juice	8	110	14
Fruit Drinks			
Orange-apricot juice drink, canned, 40% fruit juices	8	125	16
Del Monte pineapple-grapefruit juice drink	8	120	15
Del Monte pineapple-orange juice drink	8	120	15
Knudsen Hibiscus Cooler	8	94	12
Gatorade bottled drinks, all flavors	8	56	7
Hawaiian Punch canned drinks, all flavors	8	120	15
Knudsen sparkling fruit juice, strawberry	8	75	9
Hi-C canned drinks, all flavors	8	120	15
Harvest of Nature fruit punch, sugar-free	8	8	1

Drink Up and Slim Down

Beverage	Serving Size (fl. oz.)	Calories per Serving (approximate)	Calories per Ounce (approximate)
Ocean Spray Cran-Tastic blended juice drink	6	110	18
Country Time drink mixes, all flavors	8	88	11
Crystal Light drink mix, sugar-free, orange	8	4	0.5
Hawaiian Punch drink mix	8	104	13
Hi-C drink mixes, all flavors	8	104	13
Kool-Aid drink mixes, all flavors except lemonade	8	104	13
Kool-Aid drink mixes, sugar-free, all flavors	8	4	0.5
Tang drink mixes, all flavors	8	120	15
Gatorade drink mixes, all flavors	8	56	7
Kool-Aid lemonade drink mix	8	104	13
Crystal Light lemonade mix	8	4	0.5
Wyler's lemonade drink mix	8	88	11
Lemonade, from frozen concentrate	8	107	14
Coffee and Tea			
Tea, clear	8	2	0.3
Tea, instant, sweetened	8	86	11
Tea, instant, unsweetened	8	0	0

(continued)

BEVERAGE CALORIC GUIDE—*Continued*

Beverage	Serving Size (fl. oz.)	Calories per Serving (approximate)	Calories per Ounce (approximate)
Coffee and Tea—*continued*			
Celestial Seasonings Red Zinger herb tea	6	1	0.2
Coffee, black	8	2.7	0.3
Coffee, instant, black	8	1.3	0.2
General Foods International Coffee, Irish Mocha Mint	8	67	8
Magic Mountain instant herb tea	8	4	0.5
Postum cereal beverage	6	12	2
Vegetable Drinks			
Tomato juice	8	46	6
Tomato juice cocktail	8	51	6
V-8 vegetable juice cocktail	8	52	7
Carrot juice	8	93	12
Mott's Beefamato	8	97	12
Mott's Clamato	8	114	14
Knudsen Very Veggie	8	32	4
Beer			
Augsberger	12	175	15
Beck's dark	12	156	13
Beck's light	12	132	11
Birell Premium Light nonalcohol malt beverage	12	75	6
Budweiser	12	150	13
Busch	12	156	13
Coors	12	142	12

Drink Up and Slim Down

Beverage	Serving Size (fl. oz.)	Calories per Serving (approximate)	Calories per Ounce (approximate)
Coors Light	12	102	9
Dos Equis amber	12	144	12
Foster's lager	12	120	10
Gablinger's	12	96	8
Guinness Extra Stout	12	192	16
Hamm's	12	136	11
Heineken	12	152	13
Heineken Special Dark	12	192	16
Hofbrau dark reserve	12	204	17
Hofbrau light reserve	12	144	12
Kirin	12	149	12
Kronenbourg	12	170	14
Lowenbrau	12	157	13
Michelob	12	163	14
Michelob Light	12	134	11
Miller High Life	12	150	13
Miller Lite	12	96	8
Natural Light	12	110	9
Newcastle Brown Ale	12	144	12
Pabst Blue Ribbon	12	150	13
Schlitz	12	148	12
Schlitz Light	12	96	8
St. Pauli Girl light	12	144	12
St. Pauli Girl dark	12	156	13
Stroh Boch	12	157	13
Stroh Bohemian	12	148	12
Stroh Light	12	115	10
Texas Select nonalcohol malt beverage	12	65	5
Wurzburger Hofbrau nonalcohol malt beverage	12	111	9

(continued)

The Weight-Loss Guide to Food and Nutrition

BEVERAGE CALORIC GUIDE—*Continued*

Beverage	Serving Size (fl. oz.)	Calories per Serving (approximate)	Calories per Ounce (approximate)
Wine			
California brand wine cooler	3½	20	6
Carl Jung dealcoholed white wine	3	20	7
Champagne	3½	71	20
Dessert, sweet	3½	153	44
Fu-Ki saki	1½	36	24
Harvey's Bristol Cream	3½	207	59
Martinelli's sparkling cider	6	100	17
Masson light rose	3½	54	15
Port	3	134	45
Red table	3½	76	22
Sherry	3½	147	42
Taylor California Cellars Light	3½	55	16
Vermouth, dry	3½	105	30
Vermouth, sweet	3½	184	53
White table	3½	80	23
Hard Drinks			
Bailey's Original Irish Cream	1	85	85
Brandy	1	69	69
Cordials, liquer	1	97	97
Daiquiri	3½	122	35
Gin, rum, vodka, whiskey (80 proof)	1½	97	65
Gin, rum, vodka, whiskey (86 proof)	1½	105	70
Gin, rum, vodka, whiskey (90 proof)	1½	110	74

Drink Up and Slim Down

Beverage	Serving Size (fl. oz.)	Calories per Serving (approximate)	Calories per Ounce (approximate)
Gin, rum, vodka, whiskey (94 proof)	1½	116	77
Gin, rum, vodka, whiskey (100 proof)	1½	124	83
Jose Cortez tequila (80 proof)	1½	36	24
Kahlua	1	119	119
Manhattan	3¼	233	72
Martini	2½	152	61
Whiskey sour	3½	184	53
Soft Drinks			
Quinine soda	12	113	9
Club soda	12	0	0
Dad's root beer	12	158	13
Shasta root beer	12	164	14
Hires root beer	12	150	13
Old Tyme ginger beer	12	160	13
Faygo old-fashioned root beer, sugar-free	8	0	0
Dr. Brown's orange soda	12	174	15
Shasta orange soda	12	128	11
Dr. Brown's cream soda	12	162	14
A-Treat cream soda	12	126	11
Old Tyme cream soda	12	160	13
Old Tyme apple soda	12	160	13
Moxie soda	12	180	15
Yoo Hoo chocolate drink	12	180	15
Bitter Lemon	6	96	16
Pepsi	12	158	13
Diet Pepsi	12	0	0
Coca Cola	12	144	12

(continued)

BEVERAGE CALORIC GUIDE—*Continued*

Beverage	Serving Size (fl. oz.)	Calories per Serving (approximate)	Calories per Ounce (approximate)
Soft Drinks—*continued*			
Diet Coke	12	0	0
A-Treat cola, sugar-free	12	6	0.5
Dr. Pepper	12	144	12
7-Up	12	146	12
Diet 7-Up	12	4	0.3
Mountain Dew	12	178	15
Milk Drinks			
Whole milk, 3.5% fat	8	159	20
Low-fat milk, 2% fat	8	120	15
Low-fat milk, 1% fat	8	102	13
Low-fat milk, 1% fat, lactose reduced	8	100	13
Skim milk	8	86	11
Buttermilk	8	99	12
Goat's milk	8	168	21
Eggnog (no alcohol)	4	171	43
Malted milk, chocolate	8	233	29
Chocolate milk, whole	8	208	26
Hot cocoa	8	218	27
Carnation hot cocoa mix, regular	6	110	18
Carnation hot cocoa mix, sugar-free	6	50	8
Swiss Miss chocolate mix, sugar-free	8	130	16
Nestle Quik chocolate milk mix	8	245	31
Nestle Quik chocolate milk mix, sugar-free	8	140	18

Drink Up and Slim Down

Beverage	Serving Size (fl. oz.)	Calories per Serving (approximate)	Calories per Ounce (approximate)
Burger King vanilla shake	16	340	21
Burger King chocolate shake	16	340	21
McDonald's vanilla shake	16	352	22
McDonald's chocolate shake	16	383	24
Hardee's milkshake	16	391	24
Dairy Queen chocolate shake, regular	16	710	44
Ovaltine, whole milk	8	221	28
Kefir, from whole milk	8	168	21
Miscellaneous			
Ah Soy nondairy beverage, chocolate	6	149	25
Soy Moo nondairy beverage, plain	6	98	16
Ah Soy nondairy beverage, vanilla	6	142	24
Clam juice	8	20	3
Herb Ox instant beef broth	6	6	1
Herb Ox instant chicken broth	6	6	1
Mineral water	8	0	0
Pero instant cereal beverage	6	3.2	0.5
Tonic water	12	132	11
Coco Goya piña colada mixer*	3	456	154

*1 piña colada is equivalent to 3 mugs of Budweiser beer. Serving for serving, piña coladas are the most caloric alcoholic drinks in the world, tipping the scales at up to 450 calories or more each.

WALKING:
THE ANTIDOTE FOR CHEATING

Say you go ahead and help yourself to a wine cooler. Or a beer. Or another favorite beverage. You can still even the score—by walking off the calories *later*. How long you have to walk to cancel out the calories depends on the drink.

The following table shows how long you need to walk to burn off calories contained in various kinds of beverages (calculated for a person weighing 132 pounds).

Beverage	Serving Size (fl.oz.)	Walking Time
Wine cooler	12	10 min.
V-8 vegetable juice	8	20 min.
Apple juice	8	45 min.
Guinness Extra Stout	12	1 hr. 10 min.
Manhattan	2¼	1 hr. 25 min.
Ovaltine	8	1 hr. 25 min.

NINE WAYS TO CUT
YOUR ALCOHOL CALORIES

You can lose weight without forsaking alcohol completely. You just have to stop yourself from automatically drinking more than you want. Here's how.

COCKTAIL PARTIES AND BARS

Stop early. Cocktail *hour* is a misnomer—most of them last a lot longer. Set a cutoff time for yourself, or stop when you start to feel the liquor. Drink only nonalcoholic beverages after that. Better yet, schedule something for afterward that forces you to leave early.

(continued)

NINE WAYS TO CUT
YOUR ALCOHOL CALORIES—*Continued*

Switch on and off.   An alternative to stopping: Follow every drink with a glass of water. You'll always have something in your hand to sip, but you'll be getting half the liquor and calories. You'll also counteract alcohol's dehydrating actions. And a dry body is what causes the dreaded hangover.

Dilute your drink.   Start out with a regular drink, but when it's half gone, add water or club soda to it. Every time your glass is half empty again, add more water or soda.

Duck the waiter.   Never order a drink from that roving drink machine. Go to the bar and order it yourself. Chances are you'll be so involved in conversation, your trips will be limited.

Sip slowly.   A warm martini, a flat gin and tonic or a diluted Bloody Mary isn't very appealing. The longer your drink lasts, the less you'll feel like finishing it.

Fix a drink you don't like.   Some punches are so delicious that you can gulp down several glasses without thinking about it. If this happens to you, try ordering a bitter drink that doesn't appeal to you. You'll probably drink less of it.

RESTAURANT IDEAS

Dine with fine wine.   Order only one bottle of very fine wine and savor it slowly before and during your meal. You probably won't want to pay the extra expense of ordering more, and you will enjoy it more.

Order food first, drinks second.   This way, you'll probably only have time for one drink before the meal is served.

Arrive early.   Let's say you don't want to drink alcohol but don't want your friends to rib you about it. You can head these people off at the pass by arriving early and ordering a well-disguised nonalcoholic drink. If your friend wants to order a second round, you can simply tell the waiter you'll have another of "the same."

CHAPTER

16

Eat Out without Regrets

What dieter doesn't suffer from "restaurant anxiety"—the crippling fear of blowing weeks of weight control in one madcap indulgence? Well, fear no more. With a little menu savvy, you can dodge and weave your way through just about any eatery and emerge with your waistline intact.

We know. We've reviewed scores of menus from a wide array of restaurants, comparing calorie data. What we discovered may surprise you: lots of delightfully satisfying low-calorie choices (even at eateries that traditionally serve fattening fare). Our recommendations, below, are based on U.S. Department of Agriculture calorie counts for standard servings. (Keep in mind that portions and recipes do vary widely from one eating establishment to another.)

Here then, are the good, the bad and the best dinner choices for the calorie-conscious.

SEAFOOD RESTAURANT

The restaurant of choice for many dieters, seafood houses sometimes serve up deceptively fattening fare. A dozen steamed clams doesn't sound like much. But dunked in butter, they can add up to nearly 300 calories. And that's just the appetizer.

Similarly, a "low-calorie" entree like flounder stuffed with crabmeat can easily top 500 calories if it's smothered with white sauce. Beware, too, of seafood dishes with fancy last names, such as Lobster Newburg (725 calories) or Clams Casino (550). And steer clear of combination platters. These king-size dinners often feature fried fish and high-calorie concoctions such as deviled crab or crab cakes.

Better alternatives: Take tomato-based Manhattan clam chowder over the creamy New England version and save half the calories (about 80 per cup). For similar savings, choose a clear seafood gumbo over a smooth and creamy seafood bisque. Shrimp cocktail (at 100 calories for five large shrimp with cocktail sauce) is the obvious choice over steamed clams with butter. An 8-ounce lobster tail, at just 115 calories, or six steamed whole hardshell crabs, at 144, are fine dinner entrees if you can do without the butter. If you can't, stick to broiled white fish, such as flounder, scrod or haddock, moistened with lemon juice.

Best bet: "Pick and peel" shrimp with cocktail sauce. Beyond the obvious caloric advantage, any seafood—such as shrimp in the shell, stone-crab claws or steamed hardshell crabs—that you must first pry from its shell slows eating to an appetite-satisfying pace.

Our entree recommendation is grilled kabob of shrimp, scallops or white fish and vegetables at 230 calories per serving.

AMERICAN STEAK HOUSE

A juicy steak, the dieter's choice of years gone by, has fallen from favor. The reason: Many cuts of beef are high in fat, and fat is high in calories. Generally, the better the cut, the more calories from fat. Filet mignon, Delmonico and New York strip steaks owe their tenderness to fat marbling. Beware, too, steak-house toppings such as mushrooms, onions or peppers. They are usually sautéed in butter.

Better alternatives: From a calorie standpoint, London broil is a cut above the rest. At 477 calories for a generous (but often standard) 8-ounce portion, it contains up to 200 calories less per serving than the steaks mentioned above. Another calorie-miser tip: Order your meat cooked to medium-well; the longer the meat cooks, the more fat is removed from it.

Best bet: Cut your steak in half; offer the other half to your tableside partner or take it home for another meal. Then center your meal around other standard steak-house items: salad and baked potato. Ask for some low-calorie salad dressing on the side to sprinkle over your greens and potato (instead of sour cream or butter).

AMERICAN DINER

On the downside, diners tend to serve many precooked dishes, such as meat loaf and chicken croquettes, that are loaded with fattening fillers. Made-to-order items are often grilled in grease or fried.

Better alternatives: Roast turkey, at 132 calories without gravy, or broiled haddock or flounder, at 117 without butter, are standard on every diner menu. Ordering mashed potatoes (without gravy or butter) instead of bread stuffing saves you another 200 calories. For an appetizer, choose a half grapefruit or a melon wedge (each less than 50 calories) over fruit cup, which may carry the extra weight of a sugary syrup. Or have a glass of tomato juice. At 21 calories, it has about half the caloric clout of orange or apple juice and less than a quarter of that of grape juice.

Best bet: Create a 1980's grazing experience in a 1950's diner setting. Order a tossed salad, dressing on the side and an assortment of vegetables. Pickled cabbage, unsweetened applesauce, string beans, corn and low-fat cottage cheese don't add up to a hill of beans, calorically speaking. But keep in mind that pickled red beets, at 90 calories a half-cup serving, are an unexpected heavy hitter.

PIZZA SHOP

Pizza alone is not bad: about 120 calories for a slice of thin-crust pie. It's the toppings that can spell trouble. Just four slices of pepperoni double the calories in a slice of pizza. Black olives and anchovies packed in oil also carry a hefty share of calories from fat.

Better alternatives: Top your pizza with fresh vegetables, such as onions, garlic, green and red peppers and mushrooms. Go easy on the cheese and olive oil.

Best bet: One slice of thick-crust pizza, topped with all the veggies you can eat. At about 165 satisfying calories, it has half the cheese and about 100 calories less than two slices of vegetable-topped thin-crust pizza.

DELICATESSEN

Think "deli" and you probably conjure up an image of dining on the biggest hot pastrami sandwich you can possibly fit between your jaws. In reality, that can cost you upwards of 700 calories for 6 ounces of meat between two slices of rye. And you haven't tackled the "help yourself" tableful of pickles, potato salad and coleslaw! Here, lunch can easily cost you your full day's allowance of calories, especially if you splurge on cheesecake for dessert.

Better alternatives: Take a friend and share a sandwich. Then "weigh" each sandwich ingredient alone and, more important, together. At 106 calories, 3 ounces of turkey meat, for example, is the clear choice over roast beef at 150. But when the roast beef is accompanied by mustard or horseradish (each about 4 or 5 calories a tablespoon) and the drier turkey meat requires mayo or Russian dressing (100 and 75 calories, respectively), the scales tip in favor of the roast beef. Final score: half of a turkey sandwich, 267 calories; roast beef, 216. For extras, opt for pickled cabbage or a great big deli pickle, which won't cost you more than 10 calories. If you must indulge in dessert, choose a cheese blintz. Made with cottage cheese, it contains half as many calories as New York–style cheesecake (about 140).

Best bet: Half a deli sandwich consisting of 3 ounces of roast turkey, lettuce, tomato and mustard on one slice of rye (just 178 calories) or lox with tomato and onion on half a bagel (142).

MEXICAN RESTAURANT

South-of-the-border cuisine offers excellent diet fare, especially dishes that are light on meat and heavy on toppings like chopped tomato and pepper, shredded lettuce and salsa. There are two danger zones, however: fried foods and *grande* platter portions. An order of nachos (deep-fried tortilla chips topped with melted cheese and refried beans, often prepared with lard) will cost you about 800 calories. And there's more trouble in the main event: entrees heaped high with guacamole, refried beans, cheese and sour cream contain *mucho* calories.

Better alternatives: Order a la carte. Pass up the crisp corn tortillas (which are fried) and request soft flour tortillas (which are baked). Hold the cheese, sour cream and guacamole for an additional calorie saving. And, instead of the lard-laden refried beans, take a side order of Mexican rice, worth about 50 calories less. Another smart choice: A bowl of chili with beans saves about 60 calories over the all-meat chili—hold the cheese, of course.

Best bet: A soft flour taco with chicken and rice, at just 300 calories, or a light burrito (soft flour tortilla filled with lettuce, tomato, chicken and salsa), about 340.

ITALIAN RESTAURANT

From simple spaghetti houses to fine Northern Italian restaurants, one caution applies: Watch out for olive oil. A tasty but fattening ingredient (at 120 calories per tablespoon), it lurks in the garlic bread, antipasto, pesto sauce, Caesar salad, roasted sweet peppers with anchovies or tuna, and much more. Another note on fine dining: If you're intent on doing as the Romans do, be prepared for the challenge of a five-course extravaganza.

SEVEN TIPS TO LIGHTEN UP YOUR DINNER

If eating out is a treat that you don't want to give up while on a weight-loss program, here are some suggestions for calorie-conscious dining.

1. Scrutinize menu offerings with a keen eye for the two key diet destroyers: sugar and fat. Both concentrate calories.
2. Know not only what's in a dish but how it's prepared. Frying foods can double the caloric count on an otherwise low-calorie food. Fried foods that are first breaded are particularly bad: The breading soaks up fat like a sponge. If "crispy" describes an item on the menu, don't give it a second glance: It's fried.
3. Keep meat to a minimum. By nature, meat is high in fat. Ironically, diet platters listed on many menus offer the hamburger without the bun. In fact, you're better off with just the bun.
4. Don't confuse healthy foods with low-calorie ones. Polyunsaturated oils and margarine may have a cholesterol-cutting edge over animal fats, but from a dieter's

Better alternatives: For starters, choose a cup of minestrone (about 120 calories) or chicken broth with pasta (150) or an order of mussels with marinara sauce (120). Marinara, which is a meatless tomato sauce, and tomato-based red clam sauce are the lightest accompaniments to pasta. Served over a cup of spaghetti, they run about 250 calories. In the meat department, save calories by ordering chicken cacciatore, cooked in a tomato sauce, instead of chicken Parmesan, with breading and cheese. The veal dish of choice is picata, lightly sautéed with lemon. Finally, don't allow the waiter to sweet-talk you into cannoli, tortoni or spumoni. Calorie-wise, these desserts vie with the best cakes and pies America has to offer. Even the Italian ice will cost you plenty: about 250 calories.

Best bet: For a five-course meal that comes in at around 500 calories, start with melon. Next, a cup of minestrone soup, then a green salad dressed with red-wine vinegar and a fresh grinding of

standpoint, they are as bad as butter. Similarly, fatty fish such as salmon and mackerel, which are considered especially good for the heart, can take your daily calorie count too far upstream.

5. Beware the salad bar. It's the little things that mean a lot. Croutons, sunflower seeds, chow mein noodles, bacon bits and grated cheese pack even more calories per weight than the mayonnaise-based potato and macaroni salads. As for the dressings, oil and vinegar can be just as bad as the prepared blue cheese, if you have a heavy hand with the oil.

6. Pare down portions. Limit your dinner choices to the appetizers. Or order your dinner family-style; that is, one entree delivered to the center of the table from which two people serve themselves.

7. Ask the waiter if he can recommend a low-calorie offering . . . but don't take his word for it. We polled waiters at a variety of restaurants with varying degrees of success.

black pepper. Order an appetizer or child's portion of pasta with marinara sauce as an entree. Top the meal with fresh berries and a cup of espresso.

CHINESE RESTAURANT

The Chinese restaurant has enjoyed a reputation for light food. And therein lies the danger. Calorie-conscious diners assume everything on the menu is safe for consumption. In fact, fried rice, fried noodles, fried wontons and deep-fried egg rolls are heavyweights. Guess why.

Better alternatives: Choose chop suey over chow mein (which is traditionally served with fried noodles) for a 100-calorie-plus saving. Similarly, steamed rice is at least 50 calories less than fried rice. Hold the cornstarch for additional savings.

Best bet: Share an order of stir-fried chicken or shrimp with vegetables, served over steamed rice.

FRENCH RESTAURANT

First the good news: Since the French pride themselves on freshly prepared food, it's very easy for the chef to customize a dish to your diet. Now the bad news: Coaxing low-calorie fare out of a classic French chef can be an exasperating task. Fortunately, heavy cream and butter sauces are giving way to the lighter nouvelle cuisine. If your chef seems stuck in the old ways, appeal to his sense of romance: Explain that your love life is inextricably linked to your waistline.

Better alternatives: Take *salade verte* (mixed greens) over *salade Niçoise* (greens mixed with olives, eggs, tuna and anchovies) and save calories. Poached fish or quenelles (a poached fish dumpling of sorts made of pike and egg whites), or pot-au-feu (stewed chicken in broth) are excellent alternatives to the heavy, sauce-laden entrees. Know too that not all sauces are created equal: *coulis,* made of pureed vegetables, and *sauce piquante,* with tomatoes, vinegar and shallots, are calorie-miles apart from béarnaise (with egg yolks and butter), *veloute* (butter, flour and stock), béchamel (flour, butter and milk) and the crème de la crème, Mornay, made with béchamel sauce, heavy cream, egg yolks and cheese.

Best bet: Bouillabaisse—*sans aioli* (without garlic mayonnaise). This tomato- and saffron-flavored fish stew will keep you busy all night, prying mussels from their shells and lapping up every delicious drop of stock with French bread. A fabulous indulgence at just 450 calories, including the bread.

CHAPTER

17

Food and Nutrition Hints for Faster, Smarter Weight Loss

Successful weight control is, more often than not, a matter of lots of small, smart moves rather than a single, major strategy—starting with the very hardware you use to prepare food.

MAKE YOUR KITCHEN A DIETER'S DREAM

Food is tempting—everybody knows that. But did it ever occur to you that the place you keep your food could be tempting you, too? Take a look around your kitchen. The cookie jar in the corner is no dieter's friend. Those canisters of sugar, flour and cocoa that you stare at every morning over your coffee cup almost beg you to "turn us into homemade cookies."

Your kitchen need not be a standing invitation to overeat or to cook less-than-wholesome food. Here's a way to slim your kitchen as you slim yourself.

First, clear your counters of nonnutritious foods and ingredients. Next, take a look at this list of ideas on how to stock your kitchen for preparing healthier, leaner food. You don't have to spend a lot of money on new equipment, since you probably already have some of these items. You can always buy the others gradually. Before you know it, you'll have a new kitchen to go along with your new outlook on eating. These tools will make slim, healthy cooking a breeze—almost as easy as slipping on your new, slim clothes.

Blender. Its multiple functions make it practical to have on hand, especially for pureeing vegetables into "cream" soups without the cream.

Bowl of fruit. You can put this where the cookie jar used to be. If your hand automatically goes in that direction when you're hungry, you'll end up with something nutritious and low in calories to munch on.

Clay cooker. Another utensil perhaps only the serious cook can appreciate, the clay cooker allows meats to simmer slowly in their own juices, making the use of extra fats, sauces or broths unnecessary.

Double boiler. Yes, this utensil is good for more than melting chocolate. It helps warm up leftovers, like potatoes, vegetables or meat casseroles, without butter or oil. It also is handy in making the lighter sauces that are part of the slim cook's repertoire.

Egg coddler. Weight-conscious cooks know that eggs are best boiled in water, not fried in fat. Now, for an easy and tasty alternative to soft-boiled or poached, try coddled eggs. Just break open your egg into a ceramic coddler, toss in an assortment of fresh herbs and a grind of pepper, twist on the lid and gently simmer for about 6 minutes. *Voilà*—a perfectly cooked egg that's not only easy to prepare but easy to eat right out of its pretty coddler.

Fish poacher. For anyone but the true fish lover, this piece of equipment is indeed extravagant. But if you catch your own or buy fish fresh and whole, you might want to consider a poacher to enjoy your fish the way the Europeans do—delicately cooked with herbs and vegetables in a poaching liquid.

Food processor. This handy device can do just about everything a blender can do and more. It cuts, chops, grates and juliennes vegetables within seconds. Of course, you burn fewer calories chopping this way than you would with the manual method. But some claim that the food processor's fine cutting action releases juices, particularly from onions, that reduce the need for butter or oil in sautéing.

Fresh herbs. To make the most of your slim-foods cooking, keep a supply of fresh herbs on your kitchen windowsill. Dried just can't match the taste of, say, fresh basil with summer tomatoes. You'll never miss the oily dressing!

Garlic. In addition to its ability to perk up a bland dish without adding calories, garlic has special health benefits. To maintain optimum firmness and flavor, store garlic in a dark, airy spot at about 50°F.

Grains and legumes. Fill your canisters with a variety of grains. Split peas, millet, lentils, beans and a wide variety of whole wheat pastas will give you a dried-foods pantry at the ready.

Hot-air popcorn popper. No oil goes into this electric popcorn maker, which can turn out a hot, wholesome, low-calorie snack in a matter of minutes. And it takes up a lot less room than a can of pretzels or potato chips!

Kitchen scale. Is that really a 3-ounce portion of fish you're serving yourself? When in doubt, lay it out—on your handy kitchen food scale. It's a tool that's indispensable when trying to keep your calories in check. One buying tip: Look for a diet scale that's sensitive to within ¼ ounce—usually, one with a maximum 1-pound reading.

Microwave oven. Since microwaves cook with moist heat, there's no need to use butter or oil to prevent food from sticking to dishes. Microwaving also preserves important vitamins and minerals sometimes lost with other cooking methods. The result: better nutrition and fewer calories.

Nonstick pans. Today they come in all sizes and shapes and price ranges. The advantage? They allow you to sauté without the addition of any fat. Every weight watcher should have at least one.

No-stick spray. When you're sautéing, even a nonstick pan can benefit from a quick "spritz" of no-stick spray. Made from lecithin, it can "grease" a pan with just 7 calories. Compare that to a tablespoon of oil or butter at about 100 calories.

Oven bags. For use in both conventional and microwave ovens, these bags create a moist environment—without added fats—to keep lean meats and poultry from drying out during cooking.

Ridged cast-iron skillet. For flash-in-the-pan cooking without the grease, this handy tool is great for grilling boneless chicken breasts or even sirloin burgers. The ridges help capture excess fat and keep it off your food.

Skimmer and gravy strainer. To improve the low-calorie goodness of soups, stews and gravies, try these gadgets. A flat mesh skimmer easily removes cold, congealed fat from the top of soups and stews, and the pitcherlike gravy strainer allows you to separate fat from hot broth and gravy.

Slow cooker. The leanest cuts of meat often require the longest cooking. With a slow cooker you add the ingredients, plug it in and leave for work or shopping. When you get home, the meal is done.

Spaghetti measurer. Pasta is great diet food, but not when you eat it by the pound. How many times have you made spaghetti and wound up with enough to wind around your kitchen—twice? This inexpensive little device guarantees you'll cook the right amount.

Steamer. Whether you choose a simple stainless-steel basket or an elaborate multi-tiered Oriental bamboo variety, a steamer is perfect for cooking vegetables to perfection—al dente.

Strainer. Use this to rinse all the fresh fruits and vegetables you'll have on hand. In fact, you'll use it so often, you might want to have two or three—in different sizes, of course.

Vinegar. That's right, no oil. Just vinegar. Vinegar can stand alone quite well on a salad. And with the tasty variety of flavored vinegars on the market today, you might be able to find some pretty bottles to start a collection. Raspberry, balsamic and tarragon are a nice trio to start with.

Wok. Stir-frying is a great way to cook. While a little fat is required, you don't need nearly the amount that is required for pan-frying. And as your wok gets seasoned with use, you'll find you can get away with using less and less.

Wooden spoons. Essential to protect nonstick pans from scratches when you're cooking without fat.

THE BEST AND WORST COOKING METHODS

To cut fat, how you cook your food is at least as important as what's cooking. The methods listed below with three stars are ideal in that they allow released fat to run off the food and they do not contribute additional fat in the cooking process. Those with two stars are acceptable with slight modifications. A one-star rating means the method is unacceptable: It guarantees that you'll add unwanted fat and calories to any dish. Keep in mind that proper food selection and preparation prior to cooking is essential for optimum results. Be sure to choose only the leanest cuts of meat and trim all the visible fat and skin before cooking.

Baking*** A perfect method for cooking potatoes, squash and low-fat vegetable casseroles, it requires no added fat to keep the food moist; just covering the pan is all that's needed. It's also good for poultry and fish, although you might want to marinate meats with tea or juice to prevent them from drying out.

Boiling*** An excellent fat-free cooking method, boiling does have one drawback: Foods tend to suffer nutritional losses. To counter this, boil potatoes in their skins and vegetables in boilable plastic bags.

Broiling*** Broiling on a ridged broiling pan is wonderful for meat and fish fillets because it allows the fat to run off. To prevent foods from drying out, brush with juice or clear broth.

Deep-frying* This is also called deep-fat frying, which gives you a clue as to what's wrong with this method. You plunge the food into boiling fat, where it absorbs the fatty liquid as it cooks. Fat and calories can almost double using this method.

Grilling*** Indoors or out, grilling has all the advantages of broiling: Fat runs off and no additional fat is added. To prevent foods from drying out, brush with a no-oil marinade. Lemon juice, balsamic vinegar, soy sauce or mustard make exciting alternatives to the high-fat barbecue sauces that commonly coat grilled foods.

Pan-frying** This method supplies unwanted fat for two reasons. First, it usually requires the addition of butter, margarine or oil to the pan to keep the food from sticking. Second, the food steeps in its own fat, since the pan provides no run-off. To minimize the drawbacks of this method, use only the leanest cuts of meat, meticulously trimmed, and lightly coat the pan with a no-stick spray.

Poaching*** This method is hard to match. It's the leanest way to prepare fish and chicken breast while still maintaining the meat's moistness.

Pressure-cooking** The fat-sparing advantage of this method depends on what you're cooking. Vegetables, beans and rice pressure-cooked in their natural state are low in fat. Meat stews, however, present a problem since the released fat has nowhere to go but into the stew. To minimize caloric content, cook the stew the day before serving, cool overnight in the refrigerator and skim the fat off the surface before reheating.

Roasting** This method is traditional for making beef, pork, veal or poultry roast. Usually the use of well-larded meats and constant basting ensures that the meat does not dry out during its long stint in the oven. To keep fat and calories to a minimum, however, choose only the leanest meats trimmed of all visible fat, set the roast on a wire rack so the fat can run off and baste with broth. (When you're preparing meats, you can reserve the nutrient-rich stock, defat it by placing it in the refrigerator overnight and skimming it in the morning, and use it as soup or in fat-free sauces.) Vegetables such as carrots, onions and turnips can be added to the roasting rack.

Sautéing** This method is often suggested to soften onions, mushrooms and peppers as a prelude to cooking many dishes. It's also commonly used to cook lean meats such as thinly cut chicken, fish and veal fillets. The problem is that it generally takes a tablespoon or two of butter or oil to sauté. But fat-conscious chefs successfully substitute chicken broth for the customary fat.

Spit-roasting*** This is a slow-cooking method that allows the meat to expel much of its fat. To assure moistness, marinate the meats in no-oil marinades.

Steaming*** The absolute best method to cook vegetables, steaming keeps calories to a minimum and nutrients high. Steamers and steaming baskets work equally well. For peak flavor, steam vegetables lightly (they should be slightly crunchy) then toss with lemon juice, garlic or your favorite herbs.

Stewing** Also known as braising, this slow-cooking method allows the meat to give off its fat. The trouble is that it winds up in the stew. To counter this, chill stew overnight and skim before serving. Again, use only the leanest cuts of meat, meticulously trimmed.

Stir-frying** This rapid cooking method is excellent for preparing vegetables, beef or chicken. Because it's fast and you're constantly stirring the food, it's not necessary to use oil as is commonly suggested in most recipes. A well-seasoned pan to which a little water or stock has been added is all that's needed to keep the food moist and prevent scorching.

CUT THE CALORIES, KEEP THE FLAVOR

You may be leery of spending too much time at the stove for fear that you'll end up looking like Buddha's twin brother. Ironically, giving some extra time—and careful attention—to cooking will actually *save* you calories.

The basic principle here is learning to recognize the real calorie enemies in your recipes—fat and sugar—so that by manipulating the ingredients, you can reduce the calorie total of many of your favorite dishes. In some instances, calorie savings will seem small. But you may be making up to a dozen small adjustments each day and several larger ones in the course of a week, resulting in a significant saving of calories.

Look for recipes that call for fresh ingredients. When they don't, use fresh anyway. Choosing to use only fresh ingredients optimizes every flavor and texture offered in a meal. In other words, make the most of what you are eating rather than eating the most of what you cook.

When fresh parsley is listed, for instance, *use* fresh parsley. When dehydrated parsley flakes are listed, again use fresh parsley. The pungency of this herb when fresh gives life to baked potatoes, Cornish hens or steamed onions to a degree that cannot by approached by those stale flakes for sale in the "spice" section at the grocery store. The caloric difference is practically nil, and the flavor is tremendously enhanced.

Don't ignore calls for fresh ground pepper in recipes. An old-fashioned pepper mill that grinds whole peppercorns can be a great aid in augmenting the flavor of meat and vegetables. It not only tastes more like pepper than the powder that's been pulverized and allowed to linger on the supermarket shelf for months, it also adds a theatrical touch to meal preparation.

Potatoes present a glaring example of the flavor depletion in a whole food after it is processed and preserved. Mashed potatoes made from dehydrated potato flakes are a bogus form of the real thing. Both are made with added milk and butter, but with reconstituted flakes, most of the flavor comes from these two fatty ingredients alone. With fresh-mashed, you can cut down on milk and butter—and calories—and still enjoy a lot of real potato flavor.

All vegetables, in fact, should be fresh whenever possible. Home-frozen are next best; canned are the pits. And use of vegetables in soups is no exception. From time to time, a food editor will feature a "compost" or "garbage" soup stock utilizing a week's collection of household vegetable refuse, including soft spots cut from tomatoes and cucumbers or bruised brown lettuce leaves. This may be economical in dollars-and-cents, but it is a poor way to give flavor to your soup. A limp carrot or some wilted celery is okay, but in general, don't use an ingredient in soup that you would hesitate to serve in a salad or side dish.

Fresh ideas are as important as fresh ingredients. So first of all, sit down and *read* your cookbooks. Use recipes not as strict formulas but as guidelines to be improved upon. For instance, dieters have no use for recipes that call for "a can of cream of mushroom soup" as a cream sauce for vegetables or binder in a casserole. As a super-salty excuse for mushroom sauce, it will do nothing but overpower the honest, natural flavors of your food, prompting you to eat more in an attempt to satisfy your taste buds.

If your home library of cookbooks is nonexistent or inadequate, visit your town's public library and borrow two or three to get you started.

Optimizing flavor often requires less actual work in the kitchen. And the less you do to a food, the more likely it is to help control your weight. So look for *simple* recipes.

Desserts can be okay.   Thinking about dessert is a good way to begin your new approach to less-fattening cooking, because desserts are some of the foods dieters have repeatedly been told they *must* sacrifice in order to escape permanent obesity. Not so. In fact, serving yourself something special and fun after supper may prevent those late-night attacks of "I skipped dessert so this leftover turkey drumstick won't actually set me back."

Break the rule of "no dessert" by searching your cookbooks for directions on steaming or poaching fruit, such as pears baked in wine. Or redesign some of your own family favorites.

Say your family loves apple pie. Making apple pie requires that you peel, core and slice apples; sift and measure flour; cut in shortening (F-A-T); and roll and crimp the dough. If you delight in a fancy latticework cover, the entire process can take the better part of an hour.

On the other hand, just plain apples seem to be an inelegant dessert to set before the company. *Why not just bake the apples?*

Baking somehow enhances the natural sweetness of ripe fruit and still produces something warm and yummy to serve steaming from the oven. Even with a sprinkle of brown sugar or a touch of honey, the total calories per serving are not more than 100, compared to over 300 for apple pie. Furthermore, it takes just seconds to set a corer to a few apples, compared to that precious hour spent fussing with pastry dough. The saved time is a bonus to the saved calories.

Desserts are a must if other members of your family can sit down and eat two pieces of cheesecake and not gain an ounce. The seeming unfairness of that is likely to breed feelings of hopelessness in you that will contribute toward possible failure of your weight-loss program.

So we redesigned our favorite cheesecake recipe to yield nearly 200 fewer calories per serving than the original. The result not only tastes great *and* saves calories, but it gives you enough protein (17 grams per serving) to redeem it from being an empty-calorie food.

The original cheesecake had twice as many egg yolks, over a cup of sugar, twice as much cream cheese (at 850 calories per 8-ounce package) and regular creamed cottage cheese. Switching to uncreamed cottage cheese and doubling the amount still didn't catch up to the total calories in cream cheese. Wheat germ is equivalent to graham cracker crumbs calorically, and you may prefer a higher portion of crumbs. Finally, substituting fresh fruit in the topping for the cherry-syrup filling in the original lopped another 150 calories off the total.

Sensible Sensual Cheesecake

Crust

    1 cup raw wheat germ
    1 cup fine graham cracker crumbs (about 7½ crackers)
    ⅓ cup melted butter

Filling

    4 ounces cream cheese
    2 large eggs
    1 egg white
    2 cups low-fat cottage cheese
    ⅓ cup light honey
    2 tablespoons instant nonfat dry milk powder
    1 tablespoon fresh lemon juice
    2 teaspoons vanilla extract

Topping

    1 cup plain yogurt
    1 tablespoon light honey
    1 teaspoon vanilla
       fresh strawberries or blueberries

To make the crust: Combine ingredients in medium bowl. Reserve ¼ cup for topping. Press mixture into glass pie plate or lightly buttered 9-inch springform pan. Chill briefly until set. Preheat oven to 325°F.

To make the filling: Combine all ingredients in blender until smooth.

To make the topping: In medium bowl, mix ingredients thoroughly with fork until blended.

To assemble: Pour filling into shell and bake 25 minutes. Remove cheescake from oven, spread with topping and reserved crumbs and return to oven for 10 minutes.

Remove cheesecake from oven and place on rack to cool. (The center will still be watery, but will firm up during cooling.) Chill well and top with fresh strawberries or blueberries before serving.

Yield: 8 servings
Calories: 373 (compared to 555 for the original recipe) per serving (2″ × 5″ × 1½″—generous, but realistic!)

What about those recipes for eggnog pie or Sacher torte you've collected at ladies' auxiliary bazaars? Or the chocolate soufflé clipped from *Bon Appetit*? Or the strawberry chiffon pie shared with you by one of the guys in your Wednesday evening cooking class? Can they be salvaged?

Probably not. In certain cases, substitution or alteration of recipes will produce such pitiful results that you may become justifiably discouraged. Accept the fact that as long as there is a good angel in Weight-Control Heaven devising luscious low-calorie desserts, there will be a little red devil planting calorie traps like brandy Alexander pie.

THE MEAT-BUYER'S GUIDE

If you are an avid meat-eater and want to lose weight, you'll be glad to know that you don't have to scratch roasts, chops, steaks and drumsticks off your menu. While adding more fresh fruits, grains and vegetables to your diet is a necessary part of any slim-foods plan, you can continue to enjoy your favorite meats. In fact, beef, poultry, pork

THE CHOICEST CUTS

Next time you're hankering for a piece of meat but want to stay on the light side of the calorie chart, stick with the meats suggested below. Remember, these figures for the top ten are for poultry without the skin and bone and lean, trimmed, good-grade meat.

Meat	Calories per 3-oz. Serving	% of Calories from Fat
Turkey breast	115	4.9
Turkey leg	135	21.5
Turkey wing	139	19.1
Chicken breast	140	19.5
Chicken drumstick	147	29.6
Heel of round	148	25.9
Round steak	149	22.2
Beef foreshank	150	24.6
Beef hindshank	150	24.6
Chuck steak	152	26.1

SOURCES: Adapted from Agriculture Handbooks No. 8-5 and 456, and Home Economics Research Report No. 31 (Washington, D.C.: U.S. Department of Agriculture).

and lamb are all healthy slim foods; you just have to know which cuts to pick. Stick with lean meat and you won't go wrong. Meat is a good part of any diet because it is very nutritious, supplying high amounts of protein and important vitamins and minerals like iron and B vitamins. Just remember, all calorie counts listed are for 3-ounce servings, an amount that will satisfy but not stuff you.

Beef. Beef is by far the most popular meat in America, and also the one blamed most often for weight gain. Well, in some ways beef deserves its bad reputation; many cuts *are* fattening. But if you avoid high-calorie, high-fat cuts of beef, there is no reason why steaks and roasts can't be a part of your slim-foods diet. First, as with all meat, you should learn to trim any extra fat from the beef you buy.

If you stick with lean meats, you won't feel deprived. Versatile round steak has only 149 calories per serving, about the same as a chuck steak. The fat can be easily trimmed from either of these. Flank steak, which is usually lean when purchased, can be tenderized with a marinade and broiled or grilled. It contains only 167 calories.

If you feel like celebrating with a steak dinner, don't let your diet spoil the occasion. Try a sirloin steak, with 204 calories per serving, or a T-bone or porterhouse, which have about 190 calories per serving.

The best advice is to avoid any roasts or steaks that are well marbled or pocketed with fatty areas.

Avoid ribs—the meat is usually connected to the bone by a healthy portion of fat. Club steak and rib roasts are also high in fat and calories. Some of the worst offenders are chuck rib roast, with 321 calories per serving, and corned beef, which will add 317 calories to your frame.

Finally, don't gravitate toward the cheaper ground beef; it is usually highest in fat. Leaner beef costs more but doesn't shrink as much during cooking and is far lower in calories.

Lamb. Because of its expense, lamb is seen by many Americans as a special treat served on rare occasions. But the expense is well worth it if it's lean and low-calorie meat that you're after. An average serving costs only 150 calories. Some cuts are better than others, of course, and leg of lamb is at the top. A cooked 3-ounce portion will add only 156 calories to your energy supply. Lamb shank, which can be cooked in many different ways, has only 153 calories per serving. And an elegant portion of rack of lamb contains only 197 calories. In fact, lamb is an all-around good meat for weight-conscious people. The cut that weighs in with the most calories—arm chops—still has only 237 per serving.

Pork. Pork producers have responded to the nation's desire for low-calorie foods by breeding leaner animals. The results are encouraging for dieters: Pork averages only 198 calories per serving. The best all-around cut of pork in terms of calories is a lightly cured ham, which weighs in at 140 calories per serving. However, ham does have its drawbacks. For one, it's high in salt, which can make you retain water. So it's best to use such cuts sparingly, if at all. Rather, you might want to go for a fresh ham—also low in calories at 188 per serving—which has much less salt. You should also consider a loin cut of pork, at 204 calories per serving. Its tenderloin is a mere 141 calories!

Poultry. When it comes to low-calorie food, poultry is nothing to squawk at. It is one of the best all-around diet foods—though you have to watch out for a few high-fat cuts—and it's relatively inexpensive and easy to prepare. There are a few secrets to choosing and preparing your birds, however. A large source of calories in poultry is the skin, and the fat that lies just underneath. Removing the skin and fat *before* you cook the bird will reduce the fat content by almost half. For example, one whole uncooked chicken breast has 87 percent more fat than a breast with the skin removed. A whole drumstick has 61 percent more fat than a skinless drumstick. A whole thigh has 74 percent more fat than a trimmed, lean thigh. So remove the skin and remember this tip: Thighs are highest in calories to start with, because they have more fat, and breasts are lowest.

The type of bird you choose to cook also makes a difference in the calories you consume. According to Linda Posati, a nutritionist with the U.S. Department of Agriculture (USDA), "Turkey is the leanest poultry you can buy." She also says that the younger the turkey, the better: "Hens and toms are larger and much higher in fat and calories than young turkeys." The USDA rates the varying types of poultry by fat content as follows (figures are per 100 grams, or 3½ ounces, of a whole bird, minus the neck and giblets): Chicken, 15.06 grams with skin but only 3.08 grams without; turkey, 8.02 with skin, but only 2.86 without; duck, 39.34 with skin but only 5.95 without; goose, 33.62 with skin but only 7.13 without.

Judging from these figures, it might be wise to save duck and goose for special occasions. Stick to chicken and turkey, and make no bones about removing the skin.

LUSCIOUS LOW-FAT CHEESES REALLY EXIST

Blah.

That's what you have to say about that low-fat cheese you just tasted. Blah.

Being a cheese-lover and a weight-watcher simultaneously is not easy. Cheese is one of the fattiest foods around. What's a cheeseaholic to do?

Well, have no fear, because good-tasting, low-fat cheeses actually exist. You can even make them taste better. But you must have some cheese savvy. Just follow these rules.

Suit your taste.   Don't give up on the first blah. You may come to prefer low-fat cheese, just as you have come to prefer skim milk.

And search for a brand that appeals to you. We tried a plethora of

LOW-FAT CHEESES

This table gives calorie and fat values for various brands of low-fat cheeses. The numbers in parentheses are the comparable values for the aged versions of the cheeses.

Brand	Calories	Fat (g.)
Dormans		
Lo Chol (Muenster)	70 (104)	5 (8.5)
Chedda-Delite	90 (114)	7 (9.4)
Slim Jack (Monterey)	90 (106)	7 (8.6)
Heidi's Cheese Products		
Low-Fat Ched-Style Cheese	83 (114)	5 (9.4)
Heidi Ann Lacy-Style Swiss	97 (107)	7 (7.8)
Kraft Light Naturals		
Colby	80 (112)	5 (9.1)
Mild Cheddar	80 (114)	5 (9.4)
Swiss	90 (107)	5 (7.8)
Monterey Jack	80 (106)	6 (8.6)
Lifetime		
Mozzarella	45 (72)	2 (4.5)
Mild Cheddar	55 (114)	3 (9.4)
Swiss	55 (107)	3 (7.8)
Monterey Jack	55 (106)	3 (8.6)
Weight Watchers		
Mozzarella	70 (80)	4 (6.1)
Cheddar	80 (114)	5 (9.4)

SOURCES: Adapted from manufacturers' data and Agriculture Handbook No. 8-1 (Washington, D.C.: U.S. Department of Agriculture).

low-fat cheeses at the Rodale Food Center and found a tremendous variety of flavors. Kraft Light Natural Swiss and Monterey Jack were particularly popular. "They tasted like the real thing," said some seasoned experts. Still, don't let us dictate your taste buds. If you don't like one brand, keep trying.

Eat it warm. Food doesn't taste as good when it's cold. And low-fat cheese can't stand a large reduction in taste. So leave cheese out 15 to 30 minutes before serving to milk maximum taste from it.

Better yet, melt it. Melting is almost imperative if you're using one of those plastic-wrapped, processed light cheeses, in our opinion.

Spread it out. An ounce may sound like an eensy serving, but you can stretch it out if you don't let cheese dominate your food. Instead, think of cheese as a flavoring.

Slice cheese thinly. Stick it on tomato slices, apple slices or grape halves. Eat it with fresh herbs such as basil, dill, cilantro or chives. Put it on a flavored cracker. If you add such interesting flavors, your snack will taste better with less cheese. And less fat.

Cheese down your recipes. Don't let cheese dominate your recipes either.

If a recipe calls for high-fat cheese, don't listen. Use half the amount of cheese called for. Substitute a lower-fat cheese. Try low-fat cottage cheese to replace half the cheese in a casserole. Stay away from any recipe that requires cheese as the centerpiece of a dish. Instead of making cheese enchiladas, for instance, make bean enchiladas and sprinkle on cheese if you wish.

Read labels. Watch out for labels that promise "lite" cheese. Sometimes it means a lighter color. Or less salt. You're looking for less fat. So buy cheese that contains 6 grams of fat or less per ounce—the lower the better. A *really* low-fat cheese contains 3 grams of fat or less per ounce.

GUILT-FREE CHEESE SPREADS

A dib here, a dab there and a dollop or two over there. If you're talking cheese, that's usually a fast way to wallop on those fat calories.

But it all depends what kind of cheese you're dabbing. If you want a spread that really skimps on the calories, you'll have to make it yourself.

We're talking about yogurt cream cheese. It's easy to make. The traditional method involves hanging yogurt in a cheesecloth sack attached to a kitchen faucet. But you can make it with less mess if you dump a container of yogurt into a funnel lined with a large paper coffee filter. Or buy a collapsible mesh-lined yogurt funnel (with a recipe booklet) by sending $11.95 to Millhopper Marketing Incorporated, Department L, 1110 N.W. 8th Avenue, Suite C, Gainesville, FL 32601.

Either way, you spoon plain yogurt (a brand without gelatin) into the funnel, place it over a large glass, put it in the refrigerator and let the whey drip out for 8 to 14 hours, depending on how thick you want it. Toss out the whey that drips into the glass, and you're left with yogurt cheese in the funnel. Four cups of yogurt will yield 1¼ to 1½ cups of yogurt cheese.

How does it taste? Sort of like yogurt but not quite so tangy. And it's thicker, like cream cheese. It has a scant 28 calories per ounce. Compare that with cream cheese, which has 99 calories an ounce, or margarine, at 204 calories an ounce.

Spread it plain on bagels or crackers. Mix it with herbs and spices. Replace all or part of any cream cheese in a recipe with this yogurt cream cheese. Top it with toppings. Or try these recipes.

Lemon Yogurt–Cheese Pie

Crust
  8 zwieback or graham cracker squares, crushed
  2 tablespoons margarine, melted

Filling
  2 eggs, slightly beaten, or ½ cup egg substitute
1½ cups yogurt cheese
  ⅓ cup honey
  2 tablespoons lemon juice

Topping
  ½ cup yogurt cheese
  1 teaspoon honey
  1 teaspoon vanilla extract

To make the crust: Coat 9-inch pie plate with no-stick spray. In small bowl, mix crumbs and margarine. Press mixture firmly into bottom and up sides of pie plate.
  Preheat oven to 325°F.

To make the filling: In medium bowl, combine ingredients using wire whisk. Pour into prepared shell. Bake for 15 minutes. Let cool for 1 hour.
  Preheat oven to 400°F.

(continued)

Lemon Yogurt–Cheese Pie—*Continued*

To make the topping: Combine ingredients in small bowl. Spread topping on pie. Bake for 5 minutes. Chill for 24 hours.

Yield: 8 servings
Calories: 178 per serving
Serving suggestions: Top with grated nutmeg or sliced kiwis, strawberries or bananas (dipped in lemon juice to prevent browning).

Orange–Almond Cheese

1¼ cups yogurt cheese
  2 tablespoons raisins, minced
  1 tablespoon slivered, toasted almonds, coarsely minced
1½ teaspoons honey
1½ teaspoons frozen orange juice concentrate
 ⅛ teaspoon ground cinnamon

Combine ingredients in medium bowl. Store in refrigerator.

Yield: 1¼ cups
Calories: 42 per serving (2 tablespoons)
Serving suggestions: Serve as a breakfast cheese with warm muffins or toast. Mix with hot cereal. Enjoy for dessert with freshly sliced apples or fresh fruit kabobs.

Pesto Cheese

 ⅓ cup tightly packed basil leaves
  2 tablespoons sunflower seeds
  1 teaspoon olive oil
  1 teaspoon Dijon mustard
  1 clove garlic, minced
1¼ cups yogurt cheese

Combine basil, sunflower seeds, oil, mustard and garlic in food processor or blender. Process for 10 to 15 seconds, or until paste has formed.

Transfer mixture to medium bowl. Fold in yogurt cheese until combined. Store in covered container in refrigerator.

Yield: 1¼ cups
Calories: 44 per serving (2 tablespoons)
Serving suggestions: Serve with crudités or whole grain crackers, or as a topping for baked potatoes.

SUPER-NUTRITIOUS, SUPER-LO-CAL SALADS

Salad? Everyone knows it's the surefire, low-cal food, with scads of vitamins, minerals, fiber—all the good stuff!

Or is it? It all depends on how you toss it. A salad with 1½ cups of iceberg lettuce and ¼ cup each of tomatoes, cucumbers, cabbage, onions and low-cal Italian dressing is relatively low in nutrition. On the other hand, a medley of romaine lettuce, spinach, beet greens, carrots, bell peppers, peas and low-cal tomato dressing has about as many calories but 20 times as much vitamin A, four times as much vitamin C, twice the calcium and nearly twice the potassium.

So here's how to pick a perfect blend of vegetables from your supermarket or farmer's market.

Keen greens. If your idea of salad greens is a wedge of iceberg, it's time to expand your culinary horizons. Just check out the table on the following two pages to see how you can boost your vitamin and mineral intake by turning over a new leaf. If you can't decide which ones to buy, try a mix. Pick a variety of colors, shapes and textures. You can't lose with any one of these choices—1 cup of any lettuce has no more than 10 calories.

Pick some from column A. You won't want to forget vitamin A, for smooth, healthy-looking skin, sharp night vision and optimum immunity. Several of the greens in the table are high in this nutrient.

Other good bets are carrots (15,471 international units per ½ cup), grated sweet potato (13,743 international units per ½ cup), red bell peppers (2,850 international units per ½ cup) and parsley (1,560 international units per ½ cup).

High C. Sure, vitamin C prevents colds. But that's not all it does.

"Vitamin C is the only vitamin that seems to play a role in every body function, as it holds the cells together," observes Reginald Passmore, M.D., professor of physiology at Edinburgh University in Scotland. "When it is deficient, it wreaks more havoc in more places in the body than any other nutrient."

GREEN GREATS

Green	Characteristics
Amaranth greens	Bland, mild taste that combines well with other flavors.
Arugula	Sharp, spicy, mustard flavor. An interesting change from spinach.
Beet greens	Earthy, beety, chardlike taste. Best when leaves are young and tiny.
Butterhead lettuce (buttercrunch, Boston)	Sweet, succulent lettuces with distinctive flavor and smooth, buttery texture.
Crisphead lettuce (iceberg, Great Lakes)	A mild-flavored crunchy lettuce with brittle leaf texture.
Endive	An agreeably bitter taste with chewy crispness and a strong texture. Inner leaves are sweet and mild.
French sorrel	Spring leaves are lemon flavored. A good match with onions and tomatoes.
Kale	A strong-flavored green. Tender young leaves are more delicate in flavor than older leaves.
Looseleaf lettuce (oak leaf, ruby, black-seeded Simpson)	Tender lettuce with exceptionally good texture. Leaves range from smooth to wrinkled and are green or red in color.
Mustard greens	Slightly sharp and earthy flavor. Use raw or cooked.
New Zealand spinach	Spinach flavor with a sprightly herb overtone. Not related to spinach but similar in nutrients, texture and color.
Parsley, curly	Tangy and sweet. Helps to bring out flavor of other herbs and seasonings.
Spinach	Bright and leafy, sports a grassy flavor. Thick leaves supported by tough stems.
Swiss chard	Mild, spinachlike flavor.
Watercress	Small oval leaves with peppery flavor. Use raw or cooked.

Nutrient Values (per 3½ oz. serving)

Vitamin A (I.U.)	Vitamin C (mg.)	Calcium (mg.)	Iron (mg.)	Potassium (mg.)
2,917	43.3	215	2.3	611
7,422	91	309	9.5	145
6,100	30	119	3.3	547
970	8	35	0.3	257
330	3.9	19	0.5	158
2,050	6.5	52	0.8	314
4,000	48	44	2.4	390
8,900	120	135	1.7	447
1,900	18	68	1.4	264
5,300	70	103	1.5	354
4,400	30	58	0.8	130
5,200	90	130	6.2	536
6,715	28	99	2.7	558
3,300	30	51	1.8	379
4,700	43	120	0.2	330

Look for this vitamin in green bell peppers (64 milligrams per ½ cup), podded peas (43 milligrams per cup), broccoli (41 milligrams per ½ cup), cauliflower (36 milligrams per ½ cup) and red cabbage (20 milligrams per ½ cup).

Fiber. Famed for keeping your digestion regular, preventing diseases and aiding weight loss, this is the foodstuff of the new age.

Find fiber in cooked kidney beans (3.2 grams per ½ cup), chickpeas (2.8 grams per ½ cup), green peas (2.6 grams per ½ cup) and sweet corn (1.2 grams per ½ cup).

Low-calorie extras. The following selections are low in calories but also low in vitamins. For extra texture and taste, throw in alfalfa sprouts (1 calorie per tablespoon), scallions (2 calories per tablespoon), cucumbers (7 calories per ½ cup), celery (9 calories per ½ cup), mushrooms (9 calories per ½ cup), radishes (10 calories per ½ cup) and tomatoes (12 calories per half tomato).

Dressing for success. When it comes time to dress your salads, don't drown them in an oil-and-vinegar sea. In fact, you can often forgo the oil altogether for healthy low-fat, low-calorie salads. And remember, a little vinegar goes a long way. You need just enough dressing to lightly coat and flavor the vegetables. In general, a tablespoon or two is sufficient for four servings.

Here are some flavor combinations for quick-fix dressings:

- Apple-cider vinegar with freshly grated nutmeg or cinnamon.
- Buttermilk, Dijon mustard and toasted poppyseeds.
- Tomato juice, red-wine vinegar, garlic and ground cumin.
- Orange juice, rice vinegar and minced fresh tarragon.
- Red-wine vinegar with garlic, puree of roasted sweet red pepper and a pinch of dry mustard.

No matter what kind of dressing you're using, make sure your greens and other vegetables are perfectly dry. Any water on the ingredients will prevent the dressing from sticking. And it won't do you any good pooled at the bottom of the bowl.

"RICH 'N' THIN" SAUCES YOU'LL LOVE

So you've started eating poultry and fish more often, huh? Wonderful! That's a great way to cut down on fat and calories.

But if you're still pouring butter, hollandaise or creamy sauce on breaded, fried fillets of chicken and flounder, you might as well be eating filet mignon.

Instead, broil meat, poultry and fish. Or poach it in a little seasoned stock or liquid. Then, to make things interesting, whip up a low-cal sauce. Here are a few delicious sauces from the Rodale Food Center.

Cranberry and Pear Sauce

    4 pears, cored and chopped
    ½ cup cranberries
    1 tablespoon frozen orange juice concentrate
    ¼ cup raisins
    1 vanilla bean
       pinch of ground cinnamon
       pinch of grated nutmeg
    1 tablespoon raspberry vinegar or other fruity vinegar

In medium saucepan, combine pears, cranberries, orange juice concentrate and raisins. Cook, stirring frequently, over medium heat until fruit begins to soften, about 5 minutes. Crush mixture with potato masher. Add vanilla bean, cinnamon and nutmeg. Cook for about 15 minutes more, or until sauce is thick and bubbly.

Use tongs to remove and discard vanilla bean, then stir in vinegar. Serve warm or at room temperature.

Yield: 2 cups
Calories: 79 per serving (¼ cup)
Serving suggestion: This is particularly good on turkey. Try it for Thanksgiving.

Yogurt–Horseradish Sauce

    1 cup low-fat yogurt
    1 teaspoon prepared horseradish
    1 tablespoon chopped fresh dill

Combine ingredients in small bowl.

(continued)

Yogurt–Horseradish Sauce—*Continued*

Yield: 1 cup
Calories: 37 per serving (¼ cup)
Serving suggestion: This sauce has a unique flavor that goes well with fish.

Onion Sauce

   1 tablespoon margarine or butter
   1 pound onions, thinly sliced
   1 tablespoon honey
   2 small cloves garlic, minced
  ¼ cup red-wine vinegar
  ⅓ cup beef or chicken stock
  ¼ teaspoon freshly ground black pepper
  ¼ teaspoon crushed coriander seed

Melt margarine or butter in medium nonstick skillet over low heat. Add onions, then cover and cook, stirring occasionally, until softened, about 10 minutes.

Add honey and garlic and cook uncovered for 5 minutes, or until onions begin to turn reddish brown. Transfer mixture to food processor or blender and puree until smooth.

Return mixture to frying pan. Blend in vinegar, stock, pepper and coriander. Bring to a boil, then simmer 1 minute. If thinner sauce is desired, add more stock.

Yield: 1½ cups
Calories: 54 per serving (¼ cup)
Serving suggestion: Use on roasted meats and poultry.

Mustard Sauce

1½ tablespoons margarine or butter
1½ tablespoons whole wheat flour
  ½ cup chicken stock
  ½ cup skim milk
  1 tablespoon Dijon mustard
  2 teaspoons snipped chives
  ⅛ teaspoon dried tarragon

In small saucepan, melt margarine or butter over medium-low heat. Stir in flour. Cook, stirring constantly, for 1 to 2 minutes. Remove pan from heat.

Whisk in stock and milk gradually. Return pan to low heat and cook, whisking constantly, until mixture thickens and comes to a boil. Simmer 1 minute. Remove from heat. Blend in mustard, chives and tarragon.

Yield: 1 cup
Calories: 64 per serving (¼ cup)

Black Magic Sauce

- 10 tablespoons water (a little more than ½ cup)
- 2 tablespoons lemon juice
- 2 tablespoons orange juice
- 2 teaspoons soy sauce
- 1 teaspoon blackstrap molasses
- 1 teaspoon vinegar
- 4 cloves garlic, crushed
- ½ teaspoon powdered bay leaves
- ¼ teaspoon dried dillweed
- ¼ teaspoon dried oregano

Combine ingredients in small bowl.

Yield: 1 cup
Calories: 16 per serving (¼ cup)
Serving suggestion: Use in place of oil when making stir-fry dishes in skillet or wok.
Variations: Feel free to experiment with the ingredients. This version has a pleasantly sweet, slightly orangy flavor. You may want to add more orange juice or cut it out altogether or reduce the amount of soy sauce or add other herbs, such as coriander.

GIVE BEANS A CHANCE

The poor misunderstood bean. Condemned as "peasant food," ridiculed for its effect on your digestive system and even suspected of being fattening, beans have attracted a lot of undeserved criticism through the ages.

EASY BEANS

"Many people have never really given beans a chance," says nutrition expert Sonja L. Connor. There are probably two reasons for this. One is convenience. Dry beans usually require a long time to soak and cook.

Here are a few tips to overcome these problems.

If you're in a rush, buy canned beans. Just rinse them off first to get rid of excess sodium.

To have presoaked beans always on hand, soak some overnight and the next morning pour off the water, spread beans on a cookie sheet and freeze. When they're hard as marbles, transfer to a container or plastic bag.

If you forget to presoak your beans, place them in boiling water and boil for 2 minutes, then let stand for one hour, covered. Then cook as directed in the recipe.

The second reason people may avoid beans is, well, flatulence. You can overcome this problem too.

Soak the beans in water for at least 3 hours. Discard the soaking water, then boil the beans in fresh water for at least 30 minutes. If additional cooking is required for your recipe, discard this water, add fresh water and complete cooking. This ritual may leach out the gas-producing carbohydrates from the beans.

Introduce beans to your diet gradually. That way, your body will have a chance to adjust to the new digestive environment that beans create.

Well, the much-maligned bean may well be the perfect diet food.

Consider this: To lose weight, you're told to eat less of so many things. Less meat. Less cheese. Less pastry. Well, here's something you can eat more of.

Eat more, lose more.   Beans have so much protein, iron, calcium and magnesium, not to mention B vitamins, that they can easily replace meat in some of your meals. And they're so skimpy on fat, you can eat more and weigh less. For about the same amount of calories, you can eat a minuscule 3-ounce serving of meat or a 1½-cup heap of bean casserole.

And you can not only eat more but feel full longer. Beans mosey along your digestive tract nice and slowly, which means your stomach stays full longer.

Dropping the cholesterol levels in your blood can save your life. And of all the high-fiber foods that scour cholesterol from the system, probably none are more effective than beans.

Fit beans into your diet.   So what are you waiting for? If beans aren't part of your life, they should be. Feature beans in salads, soups, casseroles, Mexican dishes and dips.

Gradually increase the beans in your life to 3 to 5 cups a week, suggests Sonja L. Connor, a registered dietitian who is research assistant professor of clinical nutrition at Oregon Health Sciences University and coauthor of *The New American Diet.*

If you're not ready to eat beans instead of meat, then eat them both. Use meat as a condiment to a bean casserole. After a while, you may even prefer the bean dishes and decide to forgo the meat.

And if you do cut the meat, make sure you eat some grains such as millet, barley, rice or whole grain bread with your meal, recommends Diane Drabinsky, staff dietitian at the Rodale Food Center. Beans alone don't have the whole range of amino acids that make up a complete protein.

CREAMY, SLENDERIZING SOUPS

Soup aroma wafts through your house, filling it with homey warmth. By the time the brew is ready, you're ready for it, too. At long last, you savor the thick, creamy potion and laugh at the storms that rage outside.

Yes, soup is a perfect winter brew. It's delicious. It's toasty warm. It's even, well, comforting. It's low-fat (if you pick the right recipes). And it may act as an appetite suppressant, too.

When researchers at the Baylor College of Medicine and Arkansas Department of Health included soup at least once a day in the diets of a group of would-be weight-losers, the soup group wound up considerably slimmer after one year than a group instructed to eat the same number of calories but without soup.

Why?

Soup helped them to eat more slowly, allowing them to feel more satisfied than the soupless dieters. Other studies have backed up this theory—people who eat more soup seem to eat less food and gain less weight.

Another good thing about soups: They're easy to make, and you can improvise. But whether you make one of the soups described here or create your own, consider making your own stock. Check your favorite cookbook for stock guidelines, but be sure to trim the fat afterward—simply put it in the fridge until the fat hardens, then skim it off (imagine your body fat being skimmed along with it).

Once you have put the time and care into creating soup with a capital S, you're not going to relegate it to a role as a simple appetizer. No, this soup is meant for better things—a centerpiece of the meal. Serve it with some fresh, crusty bread—whole wheat, pumpernickel or rye will do nicely. And toss a crispy salad with light dressing on the side. Maybe add some fruit for dessert. And there you have it—a healthy, satisfying, low-cal meal!

Here are some luscious recipes to get you going.

Cream of Carrot Soup

   1 teaspoon oil
   1 small onion, sliced
3½ cups chicken broth
   2 to 3 potatoes (about ¾ pound), peeled and cubed
  ½ pound carrots, cut into rounds
  ¼ teaspoon dried thyme or basil
1⅓ cups skim milk

     In large saucepan, warm oil. Add onions and cook until brown. (Add small amount of chicken broth to onions if they stick to pan.)

     Add chicken broth, potatoes, carrots and thyme or basil. Cover and simmer over low heat until vegetables are tender, about 25 minutes. Remove from heat, let cool slightly, then add milk. In food processor or blender, puree mixture in two batches. Serve warm.

Yield: 6 servings
Calories: 88 per serving (about 1 cup)

South American Squash Soup

 5 ounces flank steak, cut into ½-inch cubes
 1 large onion, diced
 1 small butternut squash (about ¾ pound), peeled,
     seeded and cut into bite-size chunks
1½ cups pureed tomatoes
2½ cups beef stock
 ¼ teaspoon dried marjoram
 ¼ teaspoon dried thyme
 2 teaspoons soy sauce
    hot-pepper sauce, to taste

In 3-quart saucepan, sauté steak in oil until lightly browned. Remove from pan.

Place onions in pan, then top with squash. Cover and cook over low heat until onions are tender, about 15 minutes.

Add steak, tomatoes, stock, marjoram, thyme and soy sauce. Simmer over low heat until squash is tender, about 15 minutes.

Serve with hot-pepper sauce.

Yield: 8 servings
Calories: 118 per serving (about 1 cup)

Dilled Split Pea Soup

 2 cups dried split peas
 8 cups water
 2 tablespoons chicken stock
 1 small onion, minced
 1 medium carrot, diced
 2 stalks celery, chopped
 2 tablespoons minced fresh dill
 1 tablespoon soy sauce
 ¼ cup low-fat yogurt (garnish)
 8 dill sprigs (garnish)

Bring peas and water to a boil in large saucepan. Reduce heat, partially cover, and simmer for 30 minutes.

(continued)

Dilled Split Pea Soup—*Continued*

Meanwhile, place stock in large skillet over low to medium heat. Add onions, carrots, celery and dill. Cook slowly, stirring occasionally, until vegetables are golden brown. Add more stock if necessary to prevent scorching.

Drain peas, reserving cooking liquid. Stir peas into vegetables already in skillet so that they can absorb the flavor. Cook for about 3 to 4 minutes over low heat.

Return mixture to saucepan, add reserved cooking liquid and soy sauce and cook for 30 minutes. Puree the soup in batches in blender on low speed. Reheat, if necessary, before serving.

To serve, place soup in individual bowls. Place dollop of yogurt and dill sprig in center of each bowl, if desired.

Yield: 8 servings
Calories: 189 per serving (about 1 cup)

ENJOY SOME HEALTHIER POPCORN

It has been slathered with sugar. Basted with butter. Sprinkled with salt. Gunked with gourmet flavors such as bubblegum, peanut butter and pizza.

But beneath all these coatings is a diet food dying to get out. A handful of popcorn has just 6 calories, compared with 114 calories in ten potato chips and 104 in ten jelly beans. And it's nutritious, too. It contains iron to fight fatigue and B vitamins to steady nerves. Even dentists approve of it as a snack, because it's sugar free and has a mild cleansing and massaging effect on teeth and gums.

So make sure your popcorn stays low cal—make it yourself. Though popcorn is usually popped over a layer of oil, you can pop it dry. Place a heavy, deep saucepan over high heat. Add your popcorn kernels and cover the pan with a lid or screen. Shake the pan constantly, allowing heat to escape from time to time, until the popping sounds stop. Remove from heat. Better yet, use an electric air popper, which uses hot air instead of hot oil to explode the kernels.

In making these recipes, keep in mind that ⅓ cup of uncooked kernels makes about 6 to 8 cups of popped corn and ½ cup of uncooked yields 10 to 12 cups of popped.

And now for the fun flavors. Even the most unlikely spices can make popcorn come to life. Simply place the popcorn in a paper bag, add spices such as dill, basil, cumin, nutmeg or cinnamon, and shake. Experiment on your own, or enjoy some of our zesty bests.

Garlic Popcorn

2 to 4 tablespoons garlic powder
1 teaspoon dried oregano, crushed
8 cups popped corn

Lightly dust garlic and oregano over popcorn.

Yield: 8 cups
Calories: 65 per serving (2 cups)

Curry Popcorn

1 tablespoon margarine or butter
1½ teaspoons curry powder
8 cups popped corn

Melt margarine or butter in small saucepan and add curry powder, stirring well. Pour slowly over freshly made popcorn, toss and serve.

Yield: 8 cups
Calories: 77 per serving (2 cups)

Chili Popcorn

1 tablespoon tomato paste
½ teaspoon oil
2 to 3 teaspoons water
½ teaspoon chili powder
8 cups popped corn

Place tomato paste and oil in small skillet or saucepan over medium heat. Stir for 1 minute, then add water and chili powder. Continue cooking for 2 more minutes. Remove from

(continued)

Chili Popcorn—*Continued*

heat. (Add slightly more water if necessary to make a smooth sauce.) Pour sauce over popcorn, tossing with forks to dot each kernel with the rich red color. Serve immediately.

Yield: 8 cups
Calories: 59 per serving (2 cups)

Parmesan Popcorn

¼ cup grated Parmesan cheese
8 cups popped corn

Sprinkle cheese over hot popcorn and serve.

Yield: 8 cups
Calories: 79 per serving (2 cups)

YOUR ENERGY AND YOUR JUICE

"Wow, I could've had a V-8!" I'm not quite sure why the people in the TV commercials said that, but one good reason might be that they had trouble keeping their energy levels up. Vegetable juice cocktail is one of the few juices without a certain hidden ingredient that can send the energy levels of some people on a dizzying roller coaster ride.

That hidden ingredient in most juices is sugar. Natural sugar, yes, but lots of it—much more than you probably think. Just one glassful may have more sugar in it than a chocolate candy bar. And if you are one of those people who can't handle big hits of sugar (perhaps without even knowing it), too much fruit juice at the wrong time can short-circuit *your* juice.

Eat something very sweet, and your blood sugar goes up quickly, reaching a peak in about 1 hour. You may feel nicely reenergized at that time, particularly if what you ate was a between-meal snack. But for the next hour or so, it's all downhill. In response to the sugar surge, the pancreas secretes insulin, often enough to drive the blood sugar level *below* where it was before you ate anything. From that low point, it climbs to "normal" at a slow rate. For most of us, this may not cause any particular trouble. But for those who are sensitive to the ups and downs of blood sugar, snacking on sweet food or drinks may mean the periodic and sudden onset of fatigue or light-headedness.

The tricky part is that you can bring on sugar-related fatigue even if candy, cake or soda never touches your lips. That's because natural sugars in sweet fruits and juices (as well as honey) can send your blood sugar level bouncing around just as easily as the sucrose added to manufactured sweets (or your coffee).

What's even trickier is that the effect these sugars have on the body and your energy levels is influenced in large measure by the *form* in which they're consumed. The more they are separated from the bulk of fiber of the food in which they occur, the more quickly and the harder they hit your system. British scientists have found that if you eat an apple on an empty stomach, your blood sugar rises quickly, then falls to a level just slightly lower than the starting point. No big deal. When the same amount of apple is pureed into applesauce before being eaten—breaking up the fiber into small bits—your blood sugar drops lower. But when only the *juice* of the apple is swallowed, blood sugar drops *much* lower.

The snacks in the experiment demonstrating these differences were each engineered by scientists to contain exactly the same amount of carbohydrates, so that the effect of changing the fiber in the apple would be clearly revealed. Yet, the sheer *amount* of carbohydrates you consume will obviously contribute to the net effect on your blood sugar and energy levels, with larger amounts intensifying the violence of the ups and downs. Now you might not suppose that a glass of juice is a particularly potent source of carbohydrates. But a quick look at the table below, which shows the carbohydrate content of different drinks, may surprise you. Note that one glass (8 ounces) of apple juice contains the sugar equivalent of more than 7 teaspoons of plain table sugar. That's more sugar per ounce than cola. In fact, it's 80 percent more sugar than there is in a chocolate candy bar!

Keep in mind that we're just talking about the sugar content of beverages. Drinks have other stories to tell, too. Milk, for instance, offers lots of protein, calcium and B vitamins. Orange juice has lots of vitamin C and is certainly a "healthful" beverage despite its high content of fruit sugar. But if energy is your problem, you can't afford to ignore these natural sugars.

If you *are* worried about fluctuating energy levels, you don't necessarily have to stop drinking fruit juices. But you may have to use a little strategy. Try to combine your juice with a solid protein or starch food, like cheese, nuts, crackers or bread. Instead of having your O.J. at dawn and a muffin a few hours later, have them together.

SUGAR CONTENT OF BEVERAGES

Beverage (8 oz.)	Carbohydrates (g.)
Vegetable juice cocktail	11.0
Milk	11.4
Orange juice	25.0
Cola	25.6
Apple juice	28.9

SOURCES: Adapted from Agriculture Handbook Nos. 8-1, 8-9, 8-11 and 8-14 (Washington, D.C.: U.S. Department of Agriculture).
NOTE: 1 teaspoon of sugar contains 4 grams of carbohydrates; a chocolate candy bar has 16 grams.

These balanced "minimeals" may be easier for your system to handle than high-sugar snacks—or, for that matter, very large meals.

An alternative is simply to eat whole fruits instead of juices, so there is less effect on your blood sugar level. Another alternative is to drink water, vegetable juice cocktail or milk instead.

We aren't saying that all people with energy swings can trace their problem to sugar intake or too much snacking on juices. If the problem has come on suddenly, we advise some serious medical attention. Here are a few tips.

- Try to link the beginning of your problem with a change in living, eating or working habits. A new diet, for instance, or a new shift at work can both throw your energy levels for a loop.
- Be aware of the possible side effects of any medication you may be taking; many, such as antihistamines, can cause drowsiness.
- Consider any new stress factors in your home life or work. Your energy slumps may be telling you something about your emotional life.
- Take into account environmental factors such as household chemicals or working in an atmosphere that is smoky, stuffy, poorly illuminated or perhaps just insufferably dull.
- Try taking a brisk walk at the time when you usually become fatigued.

- Iron deficiency anemia usually makes you feel tired all day, rather than just at certain times. But a combination of low iron and low blood sugar may be especially damaging to your energy levels—and even to your personality.
- If the condition persists, do yourself a favor and see a good doctor.

FIERY FOOD CREMATES CALORIES

Food that burns your mouth also burns up extra calories, says a new study. After eating any food, your metabolic rate rises. But hot spices boost postmeal metabolism by an extra 25 percent, according to Oxford Polytechnic researchers.

They figured this out by feeding 12 people 766-calorie meals. The meals were the same, except that some were spiked with 3 grams each of chili and mustard sauce. Those who ate the spicy food burned up an extra 45 calories in 3 hours, on the average. Some people burned as much as 76 extra calories!

"It's an exciting observation, that hot foods have the potential for increasing metabolic rate," says the principal researcher, C. J. K. Henry, Ph.D. "But we're still cautious. We don't know if the metabolic rate also goes up after the second or third spicy meal—there may be a training effect. Also, it doesn't work for all hot spices—ginger has no effect on metabolism."

WHY FAT IS SO FATTENING

A calorie is a calorie, whether it comes from a piece of bread or the butter you put on it. Right?

Wrong, says Jean-Pierre Flatt, Ph.D., of the University of Massachusetts Medical School. Dr. Flatt has found that calories from dietary fat (such as butter) are more fattening than calories from carbohydrates (such as bread), because fat requires less energy to go through the food-to-body-fat process. While 23 out of every 100 carbohydrate calories get burned in the food-to-fat conversion, only 3 out of every 100 fat calories get expended. And that's a big difference.

In studies done by Elliot Danforth, Ph.D., at the University of Vermont, men overfed a diet high in carbohydrates took seven months to gain 30 pounds. By contrast, men overfed fewer calories from a diet high in fat gained 30 pounds in just three months.

"There's no question in my mind that fat is more fattening, calorie for calorie, than carbohydrates," says Dr. Danforth.

HOW HELPFUL ARE ARTIFICIAL SWEETENERS?

Obviously, substituting artificially sweetened foods for their sugary counterparts will save you some calories, but they won't necessarily help you lose weight. In a study of 78,694 women, the American Cancer Society (ACS) found that artificial-sweetener users (most used saccharin) were significantly more likely than nonusers to gain weight.

"Maybe [the artificial sweeteners] gave them a false sense of security, or something," says Lawrence Garfinkle, one of the researchers and vice-president for epidemiology and statistics at the ACS.

In other words, don't think that drinking diet soda entitles you to an extra slice of chocolate rum cake.

WHY SHAKE THE SALT HABIT?

Salt isn't fattening.

But eating too many salty foods may hinder your health and may even interfere with your weight-loss plans.

We don't mean to say that salt is the chief culprit in obesity. But you can gain many benefits without giving up anything when you "just say no" to salt.

The classic reason to cut salt is to prevent the life-threatening condition of high blood pressure. "Not everyone develops high blood pressure in response to salt," says Rudy A. Bernard, Ph.D., a professor of physiology at Michigan State University who studies salt appetite. "But being overweight increases your risk of developing high blood pressure. You don't want to eat excess salt and increase your risk even more."

Many low-salt foods are slenderizing and healthful anyway. "You want to eat lots of natural foods—fruits, vegetables and grains—because they're low in salt and nutritious," says Dr. Bernard. "It's the highly processed foods that are most often salty—and often fattening too."

And cutting salt has the pleasant side effect of reducing the bloated feeling of water retention. Here's how salt puffs you up: The salt you eat ends up in the fluid that surrounds your cells. But your body can't tolerate concentrated salt. So it draws water out of your cells and blood to dilute the salt, which means you get a little puffy. Water weight gain may account for several pounds. The water retention associated with salt intake isn't necessarily unhealthy. It just means that your clothing may fit more snugly after you eat a salty meal.

And if losing a few inches will make you feel better about yourself, then you may enjoy seeing how a low-salt diet looks on you.

Give your taste buds a break. Have you ever noticed how salty foods like barbecue potato chips, salted peanuts and cheese curls are addictive?

Why are these foods so addictive? It may be the tasty combination of fat and salt. Maybe it's the crunchiness. Who knows? But if you're one of the many who cannot stop after a few nacho chips, it's better not to start in the first place. If you chomp on fruit instead, it'll be harder (and less harmful) to overindulge.

Even if you're a full-fledged salt junky, you can break your habit. If you wean yourself off salt, your taste buds may complain at first, but

---

SALT SUBSTITUTES

Beef—basil, bay leaf, chili pepper, cumin, garlic, ginger, marjoram, onions, oregano, parsley, rosemary, sage, savory, tarragon, thyme.

Chicken—allspice, basil, bay leaf, cinnamon, curry powder, dill, garlic, ginger, mace, marjoram, nutmeg, onions, paprika, parsley, rosemary, saffron, sage, savory, thyme.

Eggs—basil, chervil, chives, coriander, curry powder, dill, fennel, marjoram, oregano, paprika, parsley, rosemary, sage, savory, tarragon, thyme.

Fish—basil, chives, curry powder, dill, garlic, ginger, marjoram, oregano, parsley, sage, savory, tarragon, thyme.

Potatoes—caraway, chives, dill, marjoram, oregano, paprika, parsley, rosemary, tarragon, thyme.

Soups—basil, bay leaf, chives, dill, garlic, marjoram, onions, parsley, rosemary, sage, savory, thyme.

they may eventually come to disdain your previous salty junk-food favorites.

"When you cut the salt in your diet, you gradually come to prefer lower levels of salt," says Mary Bertino, Ph.D., who investigated the subject at Monell Chemical Senses Center in Philadelphia. "It may take two months, but you start to pick up on the subtle tastes that salt masks."

So if you think you can never forsake your Fritos, try a trial separation. In a few months, you may be leaving your chips for less salty pastures.

Become a salt detective. Convinced? Great, you can start by discarding your saltshaker. Put dried flowers in it and stick in on a windowsill. Now go to your local grocer's and raid the spice section. Experiment with new taste combinations that might take the place of salt.

Still, that's only part of the battle. The visible salt you add to your diet makes up about 15 percent of your sodium intake, if you're a "typical" American. And Americans generally get up to 20 times as much as salt as they need. Many experts recommend that you keep your daily sodium intake under 1,400 milligrams.

And salt is often lurking where you least expect it. In cereal. In bread. In TV dinners. In pickles—one dill pickle has 928 milligrams of sodium! So become a salt detective. Read labels. Buy low-sodium versions of food if you can. And make meals from scratch if you can—mixes and frozen dinners often pour on the salt.

So shake the salt habit.

It can't hurt. It's not very hard. And the benefits are definitely worth it.

TWO MINERALS TO WATCH OUT FOR

With all of the emphasis on reducing or eliminating things from your diet, it's easy to overlook the fact that you may also be shortchanging yourself of some essential nutrients. Magnesium and zinc are two important minerals that you may lose while you're trying to lose weight.

Magnesium. Being fat can cause a heart attack. But strict dieting can actually *increase* that risk, according to researchers from Belgium. In fact, fasting and some low-calorie diets have been associated with sudden death attributed to heart failure.

FOOD SOURCES OF MAGNESIUM

Food	Portion	Magnesium (mg.)
Tofu	½ cup	127
Black-eyed peas, dried	¼ cup	98
Wheat germ, toasted	¼ cup	91
Spinach, cooked	½ cup	79
Rye flour	½ cup	74
Whole wheat flour	½ cup	68
Oatmeal	1 cup	56
Potato, baked	1 med.	55
Shredded wheat	1 cup	55
Lima beans, baby, boiled	½ cup	49
Avocado	½ med.	40
Kidney beans, boiled	½ cup	40
Banana	1 med.	33
Salmon, sockeye, canned	4 oz.	33
Brown rice, cooked	½ cup	28
Milk, skim	1 cup	28
Beef, lean, broiled	3 oz.	24

SOURCES: Adapted from Agriculture Handbook Nos. 8 and 8-1 (Washington, D.C.: U.S. Department of Agriculture).

Magnesium deficiency can sometimes be lurking at the heart of the problem. A magnesium-dependent enzyme helps generate the energy that gives each heartbeat its oomph, and there have been cases in which people with life-threatening arrhythmias have recovered their natural rhythm with no other treatment than magnesium supplementation. So overweight people who shortchange themselves on magnesium have put their hearts at risk in two different ways.

In a way, it's a case of which came first, the chicken or the egg? Because severe dieting methods can deplete your body of this important mineral. Diuretics such as diet pills can drain magnesium from the body. Fasting, even with mineral supplements, leaches magnesium from the kidneys.

Most people don't eat enough magnesium, even if they're not on a diet. The average intake of this mineral is only 245 milligrams a day—well below the 300 to 350 milligrams recommended by the National Academy of Sciences, which sets the Recommended Dietary Allowances (RDAs).

If you have a magnesium deficiency, you may notice some of the following symptoms: irritability, nervousness, muscle weakness, high blood pressure, convulsions, tremors or arrhythmia.

The good news is that many tasty, diet-friendly foods deliver healthy doses of this mineral. Check the table above to make sure you're getting your fair share.

Zinc. "There are some people who say that everything they eat turns to fat," says Platon J. Collipp, M.D. "Well, it could be true. And those people may be zinc deficient."

A mineral can make you slim?

Well, it won't exactly peel off your pounds. But if you don't eat enough zinc, you may not be losing weight as quickly as you could.

In a study Dr. Collipp conducted at the State University of New York, Stony Brook, a number of overweight children with low zinc levels did not lose weight at the expected rate. When he treated them with zinc supplements, their weight started dropping at a normal rate.

That's hardly surprising when you consider that zinc is an ingredient for 90 different enzymes in your body. A deficiency can mess with your body chemistry in many ways, some of which thwart your weight loss.

Consider the way your body handles glucose (blood sugar), for instance. A zinc-dependent enzyme in the liver acts as kind of a railroad switch in glucose metabolism. Called a branch-point enzyme, it's located right at the spot in glucose metabolism where one reaction leads to energy burning and the other to fat storage.

"Studies of rat livers show that when there's not enough zinc to go around, this enzyme becomes inactive," Dr. Collipp says. "The result is that glucose is shunted toward making fat rather than being burned for energy."

Zinc is also used to make thyroid hormone, which regulates the energy you burn. Low zinc may lead to low thyroid levels, which may lead to low metabolism and high body weight, according to Dr. Collipp.

Dr. Collipp also thinks there may be psychological connections in

Food and Nutrition Hints for Faster, Smarter Weight Loss

FOOD SOURCES OF ZINC

Food	Portion	Zinc (mg.)
Beef liver	3 oz.	5.2
Beef, lean	3 oz.	4.6
Pumpkin seeds, roasted	¼ cup	4.2
Cashews, dry roasted	¼ cup	1.9
Sunflower seeds	¼ cup	1.7
Turkey, white meat	3 oz.	1.7
Black-eyed peas	½ cup	1.5
Chick-peas, cooked	½ cup	1.3
Lentils, cooked	½ cup	1.3
Swiss cheese	1 oz.	1.1
Peas, cooked	½ cup	1.0

SOURCES: Adapted from
Agriculture Handbook Nos. 8-1, 8-5, 8-8, 8-11, 8-12, 8-13 and 8-16 (Washington, D.C.: U.S. Department of Agriculture).
"Provisional Tables on the Zinc Content of Foods," by E. W. Murphy, B. W. Willis and B. K. Watt, in *Journal of the American Dietetic Association,* April 1975.
McCance and Widdowson's The Composition of Foods, by A. A. Paul and D. A. T. Southgate (New York: Elsevier/North Holland Biomedical, 1978).

zinc's effect on eating. Zinc-deficient children can't seem to discern the difference between feeling hungry and feeling full.

"Quite a few studies link zinc deficiencies with brain disorders, like learning problems," Dr. Collipp says. "I think a zinc deficiency may also affect some part of the brain involved in the self-monitoring of the body, a kind of satiation center that lets you know when you've had enough to eat or drink."

What's more, getting all the zinc you need might be one way to cut down on sugar. In one study, people who received zinc supplements experienced an improvement in their ability to taste sweetness. These were ordinary, healthy people with no outward signs of zinc deficiency. That means zinc can help you become more sensitive to sweetness and require less sugar to achieve the same taste.

Aside from its effect on appetite and body weight, zinc plays a role in the maintenance of male fertility, disease resistance, brain development and cell growth. It's even been known to help reduce inflammation, reduce body odor, improve the senses of taste and smell, improve night vision, relieve cold symptoms and clear up acne and boils.

"The average American is getting only two-thirds the RDA of zinc," says Dr. Collipp. "You should be getting 15 milligrams a day."

If you're cutting down on meat, you may also be cutting down on zinc—something you can ill afford to do, especially if you are diabetic. Diabetics are at high risk for a deficiency. "If you're diabetic, you're particularly excreting excess zinc from your system," says Dr. Collipp. "And that can be serious, because many diabetics need to lose weight. I prescribe zinc supplements to all my diabetic patients."

Telltale symptoms of a zinc deficiency may include white spots on your fingernails, poor wound healing and mouth ulcers.

Convinced? Then look for zinc in meats, legumes and whole grains. See the table above to see if you're getting enough from your food.

WHAT ABOUT FASTING?

"There are no known therapeutic reasons for a total fast, not even weight loss, because the dramatic change in body metabolism it creates could cause organ failure and disease, and the composition of the weight loss would be an unacceptable amount of body fluid and tissue protein from muscles and organs," George Blackburn, M.D., Ph.D., director of nutrition support services at New England Deaconess Hospital, Boston, says.

Most of the benefits seen in fasting come from food reduction and weight loss and could be produced much more safely with a prudent diet, he says.

Fasting, like any diet where you eat fewer calories than you burn, forces your body to consume its own tissues to stay alive, says James Naughton, M.D., a professor of medicine at the University of California at San Francisco, who has a special interest in fasting.

Normally after a meal, the body uses the glucose from the meal to provide energy to the brain and other organs. It also stores some glucose in the liver and muscles.

When you haven't eaten for 12 hours or so, the body begins to use the glucose stored in the liver. That supply, though, lasts less than a day. The muscles then begin to break down their own protein for energy and to release amino acids, which are converted to glucose. This is the major source of energy for the brain and nervous system from the second to about the fourteenth day of a fast, and with it goes a large loss of salt, water and protein. (In fact, up to half the weight lost early in a fast is water that is quickly regained when eating resumes, Dr. Blackburn says.)

But as the fast and the breakdown of tissue continue, body chemistry changes. More and more fat goes to the liver, where it is broken down into compounds called ketones. After about three or four days of fasting, the body starts producing ketones for energy. The body slowly burns more and more ketones and less glucose, so that by about the twenty-first day of the fast, it's burning 90 percent fat and 10 percent protein. It continues at this ratio until it uses up its store of fat.

Then the body makes a final fatal dip into its protein supplies in the muscles and organs. Weakened chest muscles and the inability to clear secretions from the lungs make pneumonia the leading cause of fasting deaths. Fatal heart arrhythmia may also occur.

There are risks at the beginning of a fast, too, Dr. Blackburn contends. "Protein and mineral losses are front-ended. They start after 24 hours and continue for several weeks. Short fasts of 3 days, a week, 20 days, tear the guts out of the body tissue and could lead to a heart attack or stroke."

Those risks exist for someone with heart disease, artery blockage or poor nutritional status, says Dr. Naughton. "Although a healthy person seems to be able to tolerate protein and mineral losses during that time without much difficulty."

Both agree kidney stones and gout can be a problem for some fasters, too.

But some good things can also happen while you're fasting. Blood sugar and insulin levels drop, says Dr. Naughton. Although they rise again when eating is resumed, insulin levels don't always go as high as they were before the fast, possibly because glucose-starved cells have become more sensitive to insulin. But you could get these same effects by dieting off excess pounds, Dr. Naughton says.

During a fast, your blood pressure also drops, sometimes so much you feel faint. This is caused by an initial large water and sodium loss. But blood pressure quickly rises when the fast is ended, and any permanent lowering is the result of weight loss.

Hunger, the constant companion of many other diets, decreases by the third or fourth day of a fast. And the mental lethargy, apathy and irritability seen during periods of semistarvation are less prominent in total fasting, Dr. Naughton says. In fact, many fasters report a sense of well-being, euphoria and clear-headedness.

Some of these effects may be psychological, as voluntary fasters report them more often than forced fasters, Dr. Naughton says. But others may be the result of altered brain chemistry.

Both Russian and British researchers have reported that fasting raised the level of serotonin, a neurotransmitter that plays a role in mood and the ability to perceive pleasure.

But it's no magic cure. Like any other diet, unless it's coupled with changed eating habits afterward, it's notorious for quick weight regain, plus a couple of extra pounds.

"Most people don't learn much about their eating habits when they fast," Dr. Naughton says. "People who lose 50 pounds slowly on a low-calorie diet, on the other hand, can learn a tremendous amount about what and how they must eat to stay thin permanently."

Fasting's not for everyone, even its advocates agree. And it shouldn't be for *anyone* without an understanding of its risks and competent medical supervision.

WALKING WHIPS SNACKING

The next time you find yourself reaching for a sweet treat, try a brisk walk around the block first. According to a study conducted at California State University, Long Beach, a short, brisk walk will pep you up faster and keep you feeling energetic longer than a sugary snack. And low energy may be the culprit that sent you after the sugar in the first place.

For 12 days, 18 volunteers rated their energy levels before and after walking and snacking. Results showed participants experienced a brief spurt of energy after eating a sugary snack, but within an hour they began to feel even more tense and tired than before they snacked. After taking a brisk 10-minute walk, participants felt calmly energized for up to 2 hours.

But if exercise really is the most effective way to boost your energy, why is snacking the more familiar solution?

Robert Thayer, M.D., professor of psychology at California State University, Long Beach, who conducted the study, theorizes that people get hooked on sugar snacking because of the immediate energy boost. Later, they can't connect their tension with a candy bar they ate an hour earlier.

The thought of a quick trek around the block when they're already tired may seem like an aggravation, not a solution. But, comments Dr. Thayer, many participants in his study changed their snacking habits considerably once they became aware of the tension-producing effects of sugar snacking versus the calming, energizing effect of walking.

PART

III

Breaking Through the Last Barriers

CHAPTER
18

Secrets
of Successful
Motivation

Three out of four of you who say you'd do anything to be slim will fail a quiz designed to test your weight-loss motivation, according to a recent study.

That's because it's one thing to want to have a slim body, but it's quite another to be motivated to do something about it. To lose weight, you have to change your behavior. You must consistently choose low-fat foods and set aside time to exercise almost every day. For the rest of your life.

If that sounds grueling, no wonder you're not motivated! Dwell on the deprivation, and you're doomed. You'll start resenting your program, and before you know it, you'll be back to your old habits.

The only way to keep your motivation up is to make the program as much fun as possible. Remember the new pleasures you're gaining as you lose weight. After all, you're losing weight to improve your life. If your weight-loss program destroys your life, then what's the point?

So here's how to keep your motivation up and your weight down.

REMEMBER YOUR REASONS

Powerful temptations may get in the way of the best weight-loss schemes: Chocolate-chip cheesecake. Banana-cream pie. Pralines and ice cream.

In the face of these and other difficulties, you need powerful reasons to prevent you from overindulging. So take a few minutes to consider why you want to slim down. Really think about it.

"I can often predict whether or not someone will keep weight off by examining the person's reasons for losing weight," says Maurice Larocque, M.D., president of the Canadian Society of Bariatric Physicians and author of *Be Thin through Motivation*. "Some reasons can undermine your success."

So we'll help you weed out the weak reasons and concentrate on the strong ones.

Search your soul. "For my doctoral dissertation, I interviewed people who had lost 30 or more pounds and kept them off for at least a year," says Susan Ross, Ed.D., manager of the Human Resource Development Center at the College of DuPage in Glen Ellyn, Illinois. "I wanted to find out what was important to their success. Everyone said, 'This time I knew I had to do it for myself. Not for others, not for a special occasion, but for myself.'

"They said they had to do a little soul searching. Some had reasons attached to midlife. They realized they couldn't do anything about getting old, but they could do something to improve the quality of life. One woman said that she was always overweight, but she never minded it until she got pregnant and started having backaches. They were so bad, she couldn't even hold her baby. She lost weight so she could relieve the pain and hold her baby. The reasons differed—some did it for pride, others for psychological reasons and others for health, but they all had reasons that were important to them."

What's in it for you? If you lose weight to please a spouse or to become popular, your efforts may be doomed. Why?

"Let's say you're losing weight because you want to get lots of dates," says Dr. Ross. "If you successfully lose weight and you don't get dates immediately, you'll probably be discouraged and give up. You can't always please other people and you can't always depend on them for rewards. But you can reward yourself."

And though the desire to please a parent or spouse may sometimes be motivating, it may not always be that way. Say you get mad at them. Or you start resenting all the sacrifices you've been making for them. When that happens, you can kiss your weight-loss plans good-bye.

Make it positive. If you want to lose weight because you hate the way you look or because you don't want to get sick, your motivation may not be high enough.

"If you're simply trying to avoid something bad, you're working toward nothing," says Dr. Larocque. "Your brain cannot nourish itself with emptiness. If you're a pitcher and you think, 'Don't throw a curveball,' you don't know what to do instead. Instead, you can concentrate on throwing a fastball. You have to work toward something positive."

So you're losing weight. But what are you gaining? Energy? Self-esteem? Health? Remind yourself.

Keep an image in your mind. "Your mind doesn't register words as well as images," says Dr. Larocque. "So the more you can picture your reasons to lose weight, the more motivated you'll be."

For instance, if you want to lose weight for better health, imagine yourself playing ball with a grandchild when you're 70 years old. If you want to gain more energy and strength, imagine yourself backpacking.

DON'T START UNTIL YOU'RE READY

What if you don't have a compelling, personal and positive reason to lose weight?

Then don't do it. "If you're not really motivated, you'll keep losing weight and gaining it back," says Dr. Ross. "And that's not healthy. Don't try to lose weight until you're ready.

"Losing weight is a big decision. It has an impact on so many aspects of your life—health, self-esteem and relationships—it changes more than just eating behaviors. For instance, when some people start losing weight, their spouse and friends get jealous and react to them differently. Are you ready to cope with multiple changes? If you're already going through a major life change, the answer may be no."

REMEMBER: YOU CAN DO IT!

Do you believe, deep down in your soul of souls, that you can lose weight and keep it off?

If not, you may be setting yourself up for failure. "If you don't believe you can lose weight, you probably won't," says Dr. Larocque.

"If you make a mistake, you might say, 'I knew I couldn't do it,' and you'll probably stop trying."

The truth is, you can do it, even if you have failed in several attempts to lose weight. "Think of changes in your job or family life in which you've successfully gained new knowledge or skills," suggests Dr. Ross. "Weight loss and maintenance are just another change in day-to-day life that can be coped with and mastered."

Do you see your slenderizing efforts as a nasty, horrible burden you must bear? Well, no wonder you don't want to lose weight—it means a lifetime of agony! It needn't be so. A good weight-loss program isn't an orgy of deprivation.

Take a minute to write down everything that's interfering with your weight-loss plans. Why don't you want to eat healthy foods more often? Why do you dread exercise?

Now think of some fun ways to overcome these problems. Bored with diet food? Then drive to the library or the store and get a new recipe book for delicious low-fat foods. Hate exercising in front of people? Then go for solitary walks and enjoy the uniqueness of the changing seasons. Or play your favorite Broadway tunes and dance up a storm in your living room.

As each obstacle comes up, tackle it immediately. Don't take it as a sign that you've failed again. Just figure out a solution and try it.

KEEP GATHERING NEW MOTIVATIONS

"Many people gather more and more motivations as they continue to lose weight," says Dr. Ross. "People start to compliment them. They buy fashionable clothing they'd never fit into before. They feel in control and proud of their success."

After all your efforts, reaching your desired weight may come as an anticlimax. "One of the people I talked to in my study said he was considering gaining weight just so he could have the thrill of getting so many compliments about his weight loss again," says Dr. Ross. "Maintaining your weight can be more difficult than losing it, because you're not improving as much."

So add some more incentives. Have you exercised nearly every day? Then take yourself to a movie! You ate popcorn instead of potato chips at the party? Great, then buy a new record.

Treat yourself with things that make you feel good. Because if your idea of a weight-loss program means torture, then why bother?

19

Answers to Your Toughest Weight-Loss Questions

Q. I always thought that fat people had slow metabolism. But you say that going on a diet slows your metabolism down! Did I understand you correctly? And how do I get out of this trap?

A. Let's answer the second part of your question first. We interviewed Gabe Mirkin, M.D., author of *Getting Thin,* who gave us a very clear explanation of what happens when you go on a strict diet.

"When caloric intake is reduced, the body does everything in its power to conserve energy," Dr. Mirkin says. He explains that the body has an adaptive hormone called reverse T3, which goes into action when calories are reduced. "This hormone slows down the metabolism. An average 150-pound person burns about 70 calories an hour while sleeping. When he's dieting, it's reduced to about 40 calories an hour and the process is slowed down all day long. It's the body's defense against starvation."

Our approach to this dilemma is twofold. First, you are not likely to elicit a very strong hormone reaction if you reduce calories only slightly—a few hundred a day. This slower approach has another, even more certain benefit. It will give you the time you need to get used to the new eating habits described in this book. Attacking your weight problem with an aggressive 1,200-calorie-a-day diet when you're used to eating twice that much gives you no chance to learn anything and is sure to draw counterfire from reverse T3.

Second, get as much exercise as you can. Burning calories through activity does not turn your body against itself like strict dieting does. In fact, the more you exercise, the easier weight loss becomes. Greater strength and endurance make tomorrow's workout more pleasant than today's, for one thing. Then, muscle you add has a higher metabolic rate than the fat it's displacing.

Some people may find that exercise alone is the most effective way to control their weight. A hefty person who walks an hour a day will burn off about 400 calories per session. Eventually, he will walk off about 40 pounds on this regimen—assuming he doesn't begin eating more.

Q. You forgot to answer the first part of my question! Isn't it true that many fat people have slow metabolism?

A. Some do—and they tend to be people who have been fat all their lives, since babyhood. How significant these inborn traits are isn't certain.

What is certain, though, is that they can almost always be overcome with a structured approach to self-improvement. Many slender people, in my experience, have slow metabolisms. They know it and they've conditioned themselves to eat accordingly.

Q. Does it make any difference what *time* of day I eat?

A. If research carried out a few years ago at the Chronobiology Laboratories at the University of Minnesota can be confirmed by other studies, it could make a very significant difference indeed. What that research indicates, in a nutshell, is that food may be less fattening when eaten earlier in the day than when eaten in the evening.

The three university scientists (all of them named Halberg) have established quite a reputation for their research into the importance of innate body rhythms and the physiological effects of doing various activities at different times of the day. One research finding of interest to them was that when mice, normally active during hours of darkness, are permitted to eat only at the beginning of their usual activity span, they tend to weigh less than when permitted to eat only in hours of early light, a time when they are normally inactive.

Are these results applicable in some way to human beings? To find out, the Halbergs put a group of seven human beings through pretty much the same routine. In one experiment, they prepared meals that contained 2,000 calories and served them to the subjects either as breakfast or dinner. In either case, that was all they were permitted to eat the entire day. At the end of the week, the subjects who had eaten the meal for breakfast had all lost weight, while those who ate the very same meal for dinner showed either a smaller loss or a gain in weight. The breakfast-only group lost an average 2.5 pounds more than the dinner-only group.

That experiment was somewhat artificial in design, not only because the calories were limited but also because the food was selected by the scientists, and some of it was not to the liking of the participants. But a second experiment was a little more lifelike. This time, the subjects were told that they could eat whatever they wanted and as much as they wanted—the only rule was that they had to eat everything either for breakfast or for dinner. Six weeks later, after all the subjects had gone through both early and late routines, it was revealed that eating everything for breakfast rather than dinner resulted in a greater weight loss of 1.4 pounds per week.

Now, losing more than a pound a week while eating whatever you want, and as much of it as you want—even if all of it has to be crammed down in one meal—may strike you as being a very exciting possibility. It even sounds a little bit like the basis of the next fad diet. But before you get too excited, keep in mind that it would be very difficult indeed for the average person to eat just one meal a day. And before putting too much confidence in these findings, I would want to see them duplicated by scientists at several other research centers, for experience has taught me that conflicting results are more the rule than the exception.

Nevertheless, I think there's an important lesson here. And it's most applicable to dieters who practically starve themselves all day, only to give in finally late at night and demolish hundreds of calories in a matter of minutes. Not only are these people needlessly torturing themselves, they may actually be doing themselves a caloric injustice by doing their eating so late, when food might be, in effect, more fattening.

On the positive side, it might be a good idea to try to *gradually* shift more and more of your eating to the earlier hours of the day. Try it, at least; give it a chance, and see what happens. But don't try to do it all at once, because eating an enormous meal for breakfast when you aren't used to it can ruin your whole day. Neither am I suggesting that you make a meal of six eggs and four pieces of toast. Eat some vegetables, soup, stew, even meat. Perhaps after a month or so, you will find that breakfast is your largest meal of the day and lunch a little smaller, while dinner is something light, like melon and cottage cheese or even a couple of eggs and toast.

There may be a bonus in that kind of regimen, because it's been postulated by a heart specialist that eating late at night may predispose certain people to a dangerous blood clot while they are sleeping, when the fatty contents of a large dinner are absorbed into their sluggish bloodstream. It's better, according to this theory, to eat your biggest meal earlier in the day, so that when the food is absorbed, some 7 hours later, your blood circulation is relatively active and better able to cope with the sudden influx of fat.

But maybe when all is said and done, the most attractive thing about eating a greater percentage of our food earlier in the day is that, as daylight-active creatures, it's probably more *natural* for us, just as it's natural for nocturnal creatures such as mice and owls to eat during darkness.

Q. If I overeat one night, at a party, for instance, what should I do? Skip a meal the next day?

A. It is perfectly normal, and absolutely acceptable, to overdo food once in a while. By once in a while, I mean no more than once a week. Giving yourself permission to do that means that you aren't chained to a certain eating program and that you can always look forward to an occasional splurge. In the long run, it's really not going to affect your reducing or maintenance program very much at all. What's more, the less you worry about it, the more likely it is that your natural appetite control will work automatically the next day to reduce your intake of food.

Q. Is it natural to gain weight as you grow older?

A. No, it's natural to *lose* weight as you grow older. That's because our muscle mass diminishes as we grow older, so if we stay at the same weight, a higher proportion is actually fat. That will be even more true if you have not done any vigorous exercise in your mature years to try to hold on to your muscles. I know people in their sixties who weigh the same as they did in their twenties, when they were trim and muscular, but who are very obviously fat and flabby today.

Q. But don't people usually gain weight as they grow older? And is that because their metabolism is slowing down or because they are less active?

A. In America and other developed countries, there is a tendency for people to put on weight as they put on years. But that trend does not seem to hold in other countries, such as India and China. When I traveled through the Caucasus region of the Soviet Union, I noticed that the people who live to enjoy a very long and healthful life remain slender regardless of their age.

It's true that metabolism does tend to slow down a bit with the advancing years—about 2 percent every ten years—but the effect of that is insignificant compared to the lessening *activity.* The trouble is, many people do not reduce their food intake as their caloric expenditures go down. It's much better for older people to do everything possible to remain active, rather than to keep cutting back on their calories, because eventually it will be difficult for them to satisfy their protein, vitamin and mineral requirements. In advanced age, it may no longer be possible or advisable to climb a lot of stairs, carry heavy packages and do other chores that burn up calories rapidly. But that doesn't mean it's necessary to be sedentary. Walking slowly and comfortably on a level sidewalk or path will burn up those calories just the same. It may take longer, but it will be a lot safer.

Q. Isn't the high-protein diet the best way to lose weight? Many people say it is. I have a friend who has lost 40 pounds so far on the high-protein diet, and when I was on it myself, I lost 20 pounds in just a little bit more than two months—before I went off the diet and gained all the weight back.

A. No, I don't think the high-protein diet is the best way to reduce or to maintain your weight.

First, although weight loss during the first few weeks on a high-protein diet is definitely more impressive than when eating a mixed diet, it's been discovered that almost all the difference is a result of water loss. But you can only lose so much water, so eventually that rapid weight loss slows down.

There are different ways of interpreting that. Some people think it's good, because the rapid weight loss during the first month can be very encouraging. In contrast, when eating a regular or mixed diet, no weight loss at all may be experienced for the first week, because the water is temporarily retained, and that can be discouraging. (It's also one reason why I advise strongly against weighing yourself every day.)

On the other hand, what happens when people on the high-protein diet discover after two months that the same diet that was initially causing them to lose 4 or 5 pounds a week is only producing a 1- or 2-pound weight loss now? Maybe they think they're not dieting carefully enough and cut back their calories still more, only to find that the difference hardly shows up on the scale. That, too, can be very discouraging.

One of the supposed benefits of the high-protein diet is that it produces a mild state of metabolic ketosis and, as a by-product of that process, certain chemical substances called ketone bodies are created, which are said to suppress appetite. However, whether or not that really happens, or whether the effect is lasting, has now been seriously questioned.

Another theoretical benefit of the high-protein diet is that it "spares" body protein, some of which is always lost along with body fat when dieting. But that theory also has been called into question. The most recent study I've seen, in fact, reveals that eating a mixed diet actually spares *more* protein than a high-protein diet, although the difference is not statistically significant.

But the biggest objection I have to the high-protein diet is that it is *unnatural*. As you know by now, I don't believe in any diet plan that forces you to eat in a radically different manner than you're accustomed to. Eventually, either when you give up or reach your desired weight, you are going to go off the high-protein diet and revert to the same old eating patterns that made you overweight to begin with. And there is evidence that when you go off the high-protein diet, you may put your excess weight back on very rapidly indeed.

Q.   I recently retired and now at last I can get more than 20 minutes of exercise a day. I'm already up to an hour of walking with a little jogging here and there. But I feel that I'd benefit from even more. Here's my question: If you exercise for one long stretch, does that burn more calories than two shorter sessions?

A. No. With a flexible schedule like yours, the best bet is a couple of moderate-size "servings" of exercise rather than one big one. According to physiologists at the University of Nebraska, three 30-minute exercise routines burn twice as much fat as two 45-minute sets. Why? Every exercise session speeds up your body's metabolism and decreases hunger. The three-times-a-weekers gained the advantage of increased metabolism and decreased hunger for an extra day.

Q. I went to a lecture by a registered dietitian and she said—several times—that "a calorie is a calorie." Is that true? I think I've read otherwise.

A. Dietitians sometimes make that statement to fight the idea that there are magic foods or food combinations that nullify or greatly increase the "fattening power" of what you eat. While that is a meritorious idea, no, it isn't true that all calories are the same.

Here are some examples of what I mean by that.

First, calories taken in from carbohydrates—bread, potatoes, beans and the like—require more metabolic work to convert them to fat than a food that is already nearly pure fat—butter, for instance. So the "fattening power" of these kinds of foods may be substantially different than present charts indicate. In the future, we may have new charts that reflect this difference.

Second, foods with lots of fiber tend not to be digested as thoroughly as refined products. Here we may be talking about a difference of 5 to 10 percent in the number of calories you actually absorb.

Then there is the question of *when* you eat. Eating most of your food early in the day results in less calorie retention than eating the other way around.

Also, eating a really big meal at any time of day has the effect of causing more calorie storage than eating several smaller meals. Adaptive mechanisms in the body may "think" that a huge meal means you've been starving recently, and decide to do you a "favor" by turning as much of the feast to fat as they can manage.

A dietary regimen taking advantage of all these facts would emphasize eating natural complex carbohydrate foods like cereals, bread, various vegetables and beans in numerous small serving sizes, with most calories consumed by lunchtime. The opposite would be skipping breakfast, having a skimpy lunch and dinner and then busting open the ice cream locker at 10:30 P.M. In fact, many overweight people eat *exactly* that way. The result is that although their total calories may not be that much out of line, they have unwittingly created an eating style that positively maximizes the "fattening power" of their food.

Q. Which is more important to cut out of the diet, fat or sugar?

A. An ounce of sugar has about 110 calories; an ounce of fat, about 250. A tablespoon of sugar has about 45 calories; a tablespoon of cooking or salad oil, 120. On the average, between 40 and 50 percent of all the calories in a typical American diet come from fat. It's conservatively estimated (by defenders of sugar) that sucrose and other refined carbohydrates that are *added* to foods comprise another 25 percent of dietary calories.

Perhaps the best way to go about reducing the amount of fat in your diet (you don't want to eliminate it totally, because some fat is vital to health) is to trim meat of visible fat and sharply reduce the use of fried foods, butter, mayonnaise and salad dressings. The best way to cut back on sugar is to avoid cake, candy and soda pop. If you cut back on the sugar in your coffee and still drink soda, you're kidding yourself, because a 12-ounce bottle of soda contains the equivalent of more than 9 teaspoons of sugar.

Q. I went on a diet five years ago and after losing 15 pounds, it seemed like most of the weight came off my bust. My face was a little thinner, too, but there was hardly any change at all in my arms and hips. What can I do to make sure that I lose weight in the right places?

A. Have you ever heard of "spot reducing"? I've seen many articles about it in women's magazines, and some reducing spas feature it in their advertisements. But as far as I've been able to determine, spot reducing is about as real as low-cal pie in the sky.

You'd *think,* wouldn't you, that if you exercise your arms a lot, or your hips or your thighs or your stomach muscles, that the fat in those areas would be preferentially broken down to provide fuel for adjacent muscles. Only it doesn't work that way. When your body is forced either through exercise or by a deficit of incoming calories to call for fuel from its fat banks, it chooses the branch where it's going to make its withdrawal according to a scheme known only to itself. If you do a lot of hiking, most of the work is being done by your leg and back muscles, but the fat you burn up may well have come largely from your chest or arms. Or, you could do a lot of rowing, lose 10 pounds and discover that you've lost 2 inches from your waist.

You also read a lot about "toning up" this area or that area of your body, suggesting that the fat in that area is somehow either going to disappear or shrink. But I can tell you from personal experience, that doesn't happen, either. When I was 25 or 30 pounds heavier than I am now, I used to do a lot of exercise but paid no attention at all to how much I was eating. I used to do hundreds of sit-ups at a time, sometimes as many as a thousand. And my stomach muscles became hard as rocks—if you could find them under all the blubber surrounding my midsection, which you couldn't.

However, the fact that there is no such thing as spot reducing most definitely does *not* mean that you can't get your arms and hips to shed that excess fat. All you have to do is *keep* reducing until you reach your ideal weight, which would be something approximating the values found on height/weight charts. When you have reached that weight, it's almost certain that your entire body will have been normalized. Have you ever seen a person who is genuinely slender—at his ideal weight—in every part of their body except one? I haven't—with the possible exception of some women who are genuinely slender except for an especially generous bosom. It is possible, of course, that you could be reasonably slender all over except in one place, where you are *slightly* larger than normal, because that particular area happens to be the last hold-out of your fat reserves. If that's the case, the next few pounds you lose will almost certainly be withdrawn from that area.

But without exception, all the people I have seen who tell me they just can't do anything to reduce in a certain spot are substantially overweight in *more* places than that one spot. In order to trim down that one spot, they first have to get rid of the excess fat they're carrying on the other parts of their bodies.

Q. What can I do to avoid lots of loose, sagging skin after I lose weight?

A. To a very large extent, the body takes care of that naturally. However, when you lose 50 pounds or more, there is probably going to be some noticeable extra skin—although it probably won't show unless you are wearing a skimpy bathing suit. I must admit that I don't know of any exercises or special techniques to avoid that. In severe cases, plastic surgery is sometimes an option.

Q. In the community where I live, it seems that many of the women are quite a bit overweight. Most of these women have jobs, many of them in factories, and they do housework, too. You'd think they'd be burning up a lot of calories and stay slender. Why is that, or is it just a coincidence?

A. It might not be a coincidence. Researchers at the University of Michigan, who studied almost 5,000 adults in the city of Tecumseh, found that education and socioeconomic status seem to play a role in conditioning the eating habits of people. Specifically, they found that women who did not go through high school, or attended for only a few years, tended to be considerably fatter than women who had at least 12 years of schooling. But education itself seemed to be less important than economic status. There were indications that women who did not have much schooling but who married into higher-income families tended to be much leaner than similar women who married working-class husbands.

Curiously, the exact opposite trend was found in men, with relatively well-to-do men being fatter than working-class men. But the difference between women was greater, with the most educated women weighing about 11 pounds less than women with only a grade-school education. That difference is not a result of lesser height, either, because the wealthier women averaged only 26 percent body fat, as opposed to 32 percent for the less-educated women.

We can't say for sure why this trend occurs or even if it holds true in other communities besides the one studied. It's my impression, though, that it is a general tendency, and I would guess that the reason for it is simply that wealthier women place more importance on being slender.

Ethnic factors may also play a role. Some communities simply seem to enjoy eating more than others and, probably more important, do not see anything wrong with being 20, 30 or 40 pounds overweight.

On the contrary, they may believe that being well-padded is a desirable quality. A few generations ago, some historians point out, it was almost a status symbol to be fat. Slenderness was associated with not having enough money to eat well. Perhaps some people still feel that way.

None of this means that your education, wealth or ethnic origins *determine* whether you will be fat or slender. It does mean that your family, your friends and even your community can *influence* you in your eating habits. Call it peer pressure if you want to, or social feedback, or simply example. The milieu in which we live plays an important role in influencing how far we go with our education, what our aspirations are, how early we marry, how many children we have and what our life-style will be. But many people who find themselves in a given milieu simply reject some of the values they see around them and substitute their own. To be realistic, people who do this usually have a high degree of motivation.

What I'd like to say to you, then, as a person living in that community, is that you should not be afraid to have values that are different from those of the people around you and that you should make sure that your motivation is kept at a high level. It would be an excellent idea for you to seek out other people in your community who *share* your values—in this case, the desirability of being healthfully slender—and help keep each other motivated. In fact, that is a good principle regardless of what community you live in and regardless of what your unusual values may be. People who want to exercise should seek out people who already *are* exercising regularly. Probably the best way to do this is to join an appropriate club. It's a great way not only to motivate yourself but to make new friends as well.

Q.   You don't say very much in your book about overweight children. What can we do to make sure our children don't become fat or to help them reduce?

A.   The principles and techniques explained in this book will work equally well for children as for adults. Usually, getting children down to normal weight is *easier* than doing the job with an adult for the simple reason that most kids do not have the money to go into a store and come home with boxes of pastries, cases of beer and gallons of ice cream. *If you have no junk food in your house, don't use sweets as a reward and don't keep nagging your child to eat, there should be no great difficulty.* Every time I have seen a fat child, I have seen parents whose behavior needs modification, with the most common error being offering and reoffering the child food he doesn't need.

Many parents who claim that they have to buy junk food because the children "demand it" are deceiving no one but themselves: What they're really doing is using their child as an excuse to bring home junk food so *they* can eat it, too!

Other parents seem intimidated by their children and let them buy or eat anything they want. I would strongly suggest that such parents seek help from a counselor or psychologist. Or better yet, a relative or parent whose children are slim. What that friend might tell them is that it's perfectly okay for kids to squawk, complain, nag and even cry, holler and tell you they hate you. Kids act like that for all sorts of reasons. And although I'm no psychologist, I do know that the major purpose behind 90 percent of that whining and nagging is the desire to have the parent establish firm limits on what the child can get away with. Children *need* limits, they *need* discipline. They crave it; it's an integral part of their development. But there's no kid on the face of the earth who *needs* potato chips and bottles of pop.

If you have trouble handling that approach, consider how your daughter is going to feel about you when she's 17 years old and weighs 150 pounds. And remembers how you gave in to her infantile whining for sweets—which her high school psychology course will probably have taught her was nothing more than a disguised request for discipline and love.

Sure, I know that kids will eat junk at their friends' houses and can buy their own candy bars. But I doubt if 1 child in 100 is going to get fat that way.

More advice: Don't try to ingratiate yourself with your child by bringing home gallons of ice cream or boxes of snacks. There are better ways to express love. Don't urge the overweight child to take seconds or keep asking him if he's had enough to eat, just because your parents always did that to you. Don't tell the child he can have ice cream or a snack if he's good. And if he doesn't feel like eating at all or only plays with his dinner, what's wrong with that? Why not let his natural appetite control express itself? And if you have to throw out his food, fine!

Q. Isn't it obvious that if a person begins walking or doing some other form of exercise, that he or she will have a powerful desire to eat more food? So how can you lose weight by exercise alone?

A.   It may seem obvious, but it's not true. At least, for the seriously overweight.

Researchers at St. Luke's/Roosevelt Hospital Center in New York City secretly monitored the amount of food eaten by obese women (at least two-thirds over ideal weight) and normal-weight women during three 19-day phases: first a period of no exercise at all, then mild exercise, then moderate daily workouts on a treadmill.

Interestingly, the normal-weight women adjusted their diet to fit the energy demands of exercise—when their bodies burned more, they simply ate more. But the obese women continued to consume the same amount as they ate during the resting phase, no matter how much more active they became. As a result, during the no-exercise phase the difference between calories eaten and calories burned was a total gain of 11 calories a day; during mild exercise, a loss of 114 calories a day; and during moderate exercise, a loss of 369 calories a day.

Why? Rosy Woo, Ph.D., laboratory director for the Clinical Research Center at the University of Vermont, says perhaps the obese women were simply drawing on their stored energy reserves of fat during the exercise phase. But whatever the reason, those numbers would eventually add up to significant weight loss if the women were to stick to their workouts. Or, as Dr. Woo told us, "If you want to add exercise to a weight-reducing program, it would not make obese women hungrier, and it would burn calories."

Q.   My doctor mentioned to me that for some people, just looking at food can make them fat. Was he joking or was he serious?

A.   If he's up on the latest research, maybe he was serious. Although that tired old joke sounds absurd, maybe it's not.

This was demonstrated at Yale University, where psychologist Judith Rodin, Ph.D., measured the reactions in a group of former fat people to a thick, juicy steak sizzling on a grill in front of them. It was to be their reward after an 18-hour fast. Dr. Rodin took blood samples as they watched the steak cooking.

"Those who were highly responsive to the steak cooking before them also had high levels of insulin release," Dr. Rodin says. "Being turned on just by the sight of food set their metabolic process in motion. Insulin accelerates the intake of fat into the cells, so the more insulin that is secreted, the faster the fat will be stored."

Answers to Your Toughest Weight-Loss Questions

In short, those who drooled over the steak turned more of it into fat than those who didn't.

"We think 60 to 70 percent of the people who are moderately overweight are like this," says Dr. Rodin.

Q. I'm a sophomore in college. During my freshman year, I gained 13 pounds, although I certainly don't think I overate that much! Two of my four roommates also gained weight. One put on about 6 pounds and the other 10. What did we do wrong?

A. Welcome to the club. A study conducted at Stanford University by Melbourne F. Hovell, Ph.D., and associates shows that young women who live at a university gain an average of 8 pounds during their first year at school and might not lose the weight until well into their junior year, if ever.

The weight gain can be attributed to a number of causes, says Dr. Hovell. These may include suddenly changed living styles, free access to university meal-service food, communal eating, which encourages staying at the table for long periods of time, reduced activity levels and the stress of going to school in the first place.

To avoid broadening your hips as you broaden your mind, Dr. Hovell recommends trying to maintain the level of exercise you got in high school. In addition, he suggests that just being aware that people tend to gain weight during their first year may give you the incentive to avoid the richer offerings in the cafeteria and try to get all the vitamins and minerals you need in a low-calorie way.

Those who will not be living in a dorm, according to the study, have a much better chance of staying slim during college. In fact, anyone who avoids the university meal service and its unlimited seconds and thirds policy and group-gorge atmosphere—for instance, people living in off-campus housing—tend not to suffer excess poundage the way the on-campus women do.

As for the men—well, the researchers don't know. They weren't included in the study.

Q. My husband isn't making things easy for me. He keeps asking me, "When are you going to stop this stupid diet?" How should I handle that?

A. A good reply might be: "This is my new way of eating."

The worst possible reply would be something like "*You're the* stupid one! Don't you want me to lose weight?" That's bad for two reasons. First, you're insulting your husband, and that's the wrong thing for someone on a diet to do, because experience shows that support from a spouse can be one of the most important factors in determining whether or not you are successful in losing weight.

The second thing wrong with that reply is the question, "Don't you want me to lose weight?" Both you and your husband should understand right from the beginning that you're losing weight because *you* want to lose weight. Too often a spouse will reply that he or she does *not* want you to lose weight. A common remark is "I love you just the way you are!" There is a subtle implication there that he or she may not love you or will love you less if you *do* lose weight. What the real motive behind that kind of remark is, I can't exactly say, but I do know that in a great majority of cases, the initial reaction of scorn and mockery soon changes to one of new respect and admiration. And not infrequently, after you have lost a substantial amount of weight, your spouse suddenly becomes interested in slimming down, too.

But it's vital for both of you to understand that your losing weight has nothing to do with his feelings. You're doing it strictly for *your* sake, because *you* want to, because you're convinced that's what you want. But don't be too rough in getting this point across.

I like the statement, "This is my new way of eating," because it's very neutral. It doesn't make any statements about his faults, your desire to please him or anything really controversial. Further, it emphasizes the fact that you aren't on a temporary diet but that you have adopted new habits of eating that are more closely in tune with your natural appetite and your best health interests.

Q.   I've used some of the psychological techniques you've suggested, but after three months, it's becoming harder for me to stay motivated. Do you have any tips?

A.   One technique that helps many people is the self-reward system. Make a deal with yourself that if you lose a certain amount of weight by a certain date, you'll reward yourself with something really meaningful. Your goal should be reasonable, neither too demanding nor too easy. A loss of 6 to 8 pounds over a period of two months might be appropriate. If you reach that goal, be sure not to renege on the bargain. Go ahead and be good to yourself. Do something out of the ordinary. Buy some exciting new hobby equipment, a health club membership or camping equipment. One of the best gifts is new clothing, because it's probably going to be in a new and smaller size—a perfect recognition of your accomplishment as well as a reward for your efforts. Believe me, there is nothing more pampering to the ego and strengthening to your resolve than to be able to fit into a size that you haven't worn in years. In fact, you may be *forced* to be a little indulgent with yourself, because as you progress, your old clothing simply won't fit you. After you lose 20 or 25 pounds, you may well find that even your shoes are too big for you.

In my own case, my trouser size went from a 36 to a 31, my shoe size from a 9 to 8½, my sport shirt size from a medium to a small and my dress shirt from a 16 to 15½, which has to be cut full-trim to fit me. That can be an expensive proposition, but the boost to your motivation when you see how good all that new clothing looks on you is well worth it.

It's also helpful to realize that in the course of losing weight, it's perfectly natural for you to hit a plateau every now and then. There were many weeks when I thought I was following my program fairly well, but my weekly weigh-in showed no progress. I told myself that the important thing was to follow the program, not to play games with the scale. And I usually found that the next week or sometimes the week after that, I would suddenly lose 4 or 5 pounds, even though I hadn't done anything different. The name of that game is water retention, not willpower, so don't let it discourage you. That's why I advise against getting weighed more than once a week and against setting short-term weight-loss goals.

Another good way to keep up your motivation is to get more exercise. This afternoon I took a long, slow walk through the park to admire the fall foliage, and then through the prettiest section of town to admire the homes and landscaping. I didn't work up a drop of sweat, but that walk made me feel *good*—fit, relaxed and pleased with myself. The fact that it burned up hundreds of calories and actually reduced my appetite for dinner wasn't as important as the psychological effect. Taking long walks is a very obvious physical way of reminding yourself that you are a new person, a very fit and active new person.

Q. I've lost 22 pounds and I'm very happy about it, but lately I notice that I've been waking up earlier than usual, about 6:15 or 6:30 instead of 7:00 A.M. That doesn't really bother me, but I wonder about it. Is it good, bad or just a coincidence?

A. More than likely, it's simply because when you lose weight, you require less sleep. That has been shown in scientific studies, and it was also true in my case. Why heavier people require more sleep is not understood, but we can speculate that the less body mass that has to be restored and refreshed, the less time is required to do the job.

Q. Does losing weight affect your sex life?

A. It certainly *can,* either positively or negatively.

If crash-dieting leaves you feeling tired and irritable, it's obviously going to have an undesirable effect on your sex life. And not just for physical reasons but also because your irritability may alienate your spouse and strain *all* aspects of your relationship. Losing weight sensibly, however, can only help your love life. You are bound to have more energy. You will even require less sleep. You will also look better—and feel better about how you look.

Recently there have been indications that dieting can in some cases increase a man's level of testosterone, the male hormone. Men who are quite obese often have elevated levels of the female hormone estrone, which is created from a precursor in fatty tissue. Estrone is believed to suppress production of testosterone in the testicles. In one recent experiment, dieting reduced the level of estrone in 15 obese men to normal and caused an increase of testosterone to the normal level in all except 2. The men in this experiment lost an average of 45 pounds and were on a diet severely restricted to only 320 calories a day, so it isn't possible to say to what extent these findings would be applicable to all overweight men who reduce.

Q. I have gone on a diet several times, and it wasn't all that difficult for me to stick to it, even though I was only eating 1,200 calories a day. But what I *couldn't* do was keep the weight off after I'd lost it. Why was that? Shouldn't it be the other way around?

A. During the *reducing* phase of your diet, you were eating less than you were permitted to eat during the maintenance phase that followed. But even though you were eating less, your motivation was probably at a very high level and you were extremely conscious of what you were eating. You had a kind of temporary obsession, really. When we are in that kind of state, we can draw on enormous reserves of energy.

There is also a strong sense of purpose to what we are doing, and we feel ready to sacrifice almost anything in order to reach our goal.

But what happens once that goal has been reached, when you have lost your 20 or 30 or 50 pounds at the end of your diet? Suddenly there no longer seems to be a sense of purpose to your eating behavior other than enjoyment. While losing weight seems to be something positive, maintaining your weight is somehow negative and rather dull. So your sense of purpose and motivation can disappear almost overnight.

Another factor is the tendency toward a big let-down after any concentrated period of effort: physical, mental or emotional. Whether you have been dieting, studying for finals or redecorating your house, once the big burst is over, the big poop-out begins.

Add to all of the above the fact that when you are on a strict diet, you're also building up feelings of deprivation, and you can see why the "success" you had in crash-dieting (that's what a 1,200-calorie diet is, really) could not be maintained over the long haul.

I think we can all see from the above why it is wrong—so *absolutely wrong*—to set out on a weight-reduction plan with the idea in mind that your problem is that you're "X" pounds too heavy and that success will have been reached when you lose "X" pounds. That kind of thinking practically ensures that you'll regain much of what you lost. If, on the other hand, you have a very clear idea that your goal is to *change your behavior,* and in so doing lose weight naturally, there is no big poop-out.

Q. Someone told me that you can drink all the alcohol you want and never get fat, because your body can't turn alcohol into fat. That sounds ridiculous, but he insisted that he was right.

A. He *was* right—but only partly. Yes, it's true that the body cannot convert the calories in alcohol into fat. All it can do is "burn" those calories for metabolic energy. But your friend is dead wrong in asserting that you can drink all you want without getting fat. Here's why.

When your body begins burning alcohol as fuel, it *stops* burning its normal fuel. The result is that ingested food calories that would ordinarily be burned to keep you breathing and moving are stored away as fat. A few drinks before dinner and a few after are more than enough to ensure that your entire dinner will be banked as blubber. On the other hand, it does seem that alcohol is converted to energy rather inefficiently. The calories contributed may be less than the charts suggest. How much less, we can't say at this point.

Q. Is it possible that doing exercise can make you *gain* weight? I read that muscle weighs more than fat.

A. It's true that a handful of muscle weighs more than the same handful of fat, but there's no way you're going to add that much muscle to your body in the course of losing a handful of fat. Young men can add muscle mass quite readily; older men more slowly. Young women, no matter how much they exercise, even if they lift weights, cannot bulk up their bodies with muscle as much as their male counterparts can; it's a matter of hormones. And older women will add even less muscle mass. Strength, most definitely, but not bulk.

Q. If I'm not mistaken, you didn't say to check with your doctor before going on a diet. Is there a reason, or did you just forget?

A. It would be easy for me to say, "Check with your doctor before beginning any diet," which is what everyone else seems to say, and then wash my hands of any misfortune that may befall you. But in all sincerity, if you are substantially overweight—25 pounds or more—it is, at least in my opinion, much more important for you to go to your doctor and ask his permission to keep doing nothing. By doing nothing, you may well be increasing your chances of developing heart disease, high blood pressure, diabetes, arthritis, gout, low back problems or problems with your feet. By following the reducing program outlined in this book, which involves losing no more than 5 or 6 pounds a month and does not involve the elimination of any class of foods, not even junk food, it is extremely unlikely that you will be endangering your health.

On the other hand, if you are thinking of launching into one of the traditional diet plans, which usually involve eating between 800 and 1,200 calories a day, you *should* seek medical advice before doing so, as that caloric intake may represent a drastic and sudden change for you. Ironically, if you do go to a doctor to seek advice about dieting, it's likely that he will recommend that very sort of diet.

Having said that, I will back off a little and suggest that if you have a chronic metabolic disorder, such as diabetes or gout, you should not only check in with your doctor before beginning a reducing program but also keep in touch with him as things progress. You will be told, for instance, that if you have gout and go on a crash diet, you may suffer severe pain for the first few weeks as uric acid crystals are suddenly liberated. And if you have maturity-onset diabetes and are on insulin, your insulin requirements will probably be reduced as you lose weight. Many people with that form of diabetes find they can go off the hormone supplements completely when they have normalized their weight. But it is important to take neither too much nor too little insulin, so your condition should be monitored regularly.

Q. What about kneading your fat to loosen it, so that you lose it faster?

A. That seems to be a fairly well-established belief, although it's fading rapidly. And it should fade, because as far as I know, there's nothing to it. By shaking your fat, pounding it, rolling it, slapping it or thumping it, about the only thing you will accomplish is to rupture some blood vessels. If you are extremely overweight or prone to circulatory problems, you might even do worse.

The one thing you *can* do to encourage your body to burn fat is to exercise regularly. Active people burn fat much more readily than sedentary people.

Q. Many doctors say that even when you're dieting, you don't need vitamin supplements. They claim that unless your own doctor recommends them, vitamins are a waste of money. Could you explain again why you recommend supplements?

A. Deciding how you should spend your energy in the pursuit and protection of health and well-being is a very interesting process. And money is simply another form of energy, representing work you have already done, which has now been "translated" into an extraordinarily flexible, exchangeable form.

Your question has led me to calculate that during the last 15 years or so, I have spent approximately $3,500 on life insurance premiums. Having just checked my pulse, I suddenly realize that all that money has been totally wasted (plus another good chunk I could have earned in interest). Or has it?

That is not really an impertinent question, because speaking "scientifically," it *has* been wasted. And what about my health insurance policy? My property insurance? My automobile liability insurance? My special travel coverage? What about my smoke detector? My burglar-resistant lock? I'd be hard-pressed to demonstrate that those cash outlays weren't "wasted," too.

So you see, most of us spend considerable portions of our precious energy in efforts to protect ourselves (and our families) against a whole array of potential dangers, and using nutritional supplements as a kind of health insurance is just one more way in which we do this. No doctor can justifiably make the statement in print or on TV that *you* do not need supplements, any more than a financial adviser writing in a newspaper can tell *you* how much insurance you need. If either of those experts were to meet you personally and spend considerable time examining your special needs, he could give you some potentially very useful advice, although he still couldn't give *answers*. Quite possibly, *you* put a higher value on your own health or peace of mind than the experts do. And if you are highly concerned about your present and future health, you might want to not only take some supplements but also do regular exercise, avoid food additives, drink purified water and so forth. None of these things has ever been "proved" to prevent illness or lengthen your life, but there's no incontestable proof that any other program of self-protection or self-improvement is guaranteed to pay off, either.

All of the above constitutes a kind of philosophical answer to your question. The physical or biochemical part is, I hope, adequately dealt with in the main text. Keep in mind, though, that my attitude toward the need for nutritional insurance is influenced by the observation that the great majority of people who want to lose weight have a history of crash dieting. And because they are relatively sedentary, the total amount of food they can eat is quite limited. In the process of shortchanging themselves calorically, they can come very close to shortchanging themselves of vitamins and minerals as well.

CHAPTER

20

How to Lose Those Last 10 Stubborn Pounds— Forever!

Nearly everyone's got 'em. Stubborn pounds. The kind that quietly creep up over the years and seemingly settle in for life. Diet-resistant, they hang on after the other unwanted pounds have gone. And once pried from your frame, they are almost certain to return as quickly as they came off. To make matters worse, it's usually the last 10 pounds that put you within striking distance of your weight goal that are least likely to surrender without a fight.

But why should the last 10 be any tougher to shed than the first?

"I'll give you three simple reasons," says Theodore Van Itallie, M.D., co-director of the Division of Metabolism and Nutrition at St. Luke's/Roosevelt Hospital in New York City. "First, fatter people tend to have higher energy requirements. As you lose weight, you burn fewer calories just by virtue of the fact that you've become smaller and are carrying around less weight. Second, heavy people tend to be waterlogged, and water loss is the first thing to show up on the scale. Third, as you lose weight, your metabolic rate slows down."

Rapid weight loss and weight cycling—rapid weight loss followed by rapid weight gain—exacerbate the problem. Eating too little can sometimes sabotage your weight-loss efforts, Dr. Van Itallie explains. When denied food, the body feeds off the protein in muscle. And since muscle is the body's most metabolically active tissue, depleting it can reduce your body's calorie-burning ability.

CRASH DIETING CAN BE SELF-DEFEATING

Further, according to George L. Blackburn, M.D., Ph.D., director of nutrition support services at New England Deaconess Hospital in Boston, and a leading authority on weight loss, a severely restricted diet trains the body to be more energy efficient—that is, to conserve calories by slowing its resting metabolic rate. This, he says, makes it increasingly difficult to continue losing weight, and much easier to gain it back, since the metabolism usually stays depressed even after normal eating patterns resume.

Regained weight is especially stubborn. The problem is, crash dieting not only depletes muscle mass, it also promotes fat storage later, after you've gone off the diet. So pounds lost as muscle are often regained as fat. Preliminary studies have shown that as weight loss/gain cycling progresses (and the body's percentage of fat may increase), weight loss occurs more slowly and regain occurs more rapidly. "This may be why losing becomes more difficult as we get older. The body learns from many bouts of dieting, and stores fat in preparation for another shortage," says Kelly Brownell, Ph.D., co-director of the Obesity Research Center at the University of Pennsylvania School of Medicine, Philadelphia.

Still, diet-mongers insist that the more resistant the weight problem, the more drastic the measures required to resolve it. The experts we interviewed disagree with that: Stubborn pounds, they say, eventually yield to gentle persuasion. The person who takes a slow and steady approach may have a much better chance of dropping those last 10 pounds permanently.

Their general advice: Forget about extremely restricted diets or strenuous exercise regimens. What's required is patience and commitment. Don't tackle a tough weight problem unless you are quite motivated and are certain that you can stick with the kind of life-style changes mentioned below—not just till you've shed the 10 pounds, but forever, for the rest of your life.

"Look at it this way," says Dr. Van Itallie. "You can lose weight by moving from New York City to Bangladesh for two months. But when you move back to New York City you'll gain it right back. The key is to learn to live in your New York environment at a different level of energy intake and expenditure—at a different calorie economy."

So, if you are motivated and committed, then our panel of experts is ready to share with you their strategies for permanent weight loss. We presented three common "stubborn-pound" scenarios to Dr. Van Itallie, Dr. Blackburn and Dr. Brownell. Here are their recommendations for each.

Suppose, over the last five years, your weight has stabilized at a level 10 pounds above your ideal. You eat sensibly, consuming about 1,600 to 1,800 calories a day, and exercise regularly—30 minutes, three times a week. How can you safely shed those 10 pounds and maintain the lower weight?

"The best way to lose fat and retain lean muscle mass is to lose weight slowly. You can do this by reducing caloric intake by about 500 calories per day and gradually increasing caloric expenditure through exercise," says Dr. Van Itallie. "Safe weight loss occurs at an average rate of 1 percent of body weight per week. If you weigh 150 pounds, for example, aim for a loss of about 1.5 pounds a week, no more."

Dr. Blackburn's advice is similar. "If you've got 10 pounds to lose, give it a full ten weeks," he says. "In the first three to four weeks, you can expect to lose half the weight. In the next four weeks, you lose a pound a week. And in the last two weeks you'll shape up and lose more fat.

"Keep in mind that your ideal weight is one you can maintain without being hungry while eating three natural meals a day," he adds. "So don't starve yourself. Eat. Just pare down your diet to the essentials—the raw materials. Whole wheat bread. Pasta. Rice. Fruits and vegetables. Skim milk. Fish and skinless chicken. No mixed dishes. No goulash. No lasagna."

By eating a "raw-materials diet," as Dr. Blackburn calls it, you consume more complex carbohydrates and less fat. The most obvious advantage of this diet is that it satisfies by providing bulk. More important, it gives your weight-loss program a metabolic edge.

Calories from fat are metabolized quickly and efficiently. In other words, it takes very little energy to transform butter into body fat. Calories from carbohydrates present the body with a greater challenge.

It takes about five times as much energy to store the calories from, say bread, as it does from butter.

"You have to make a distinction between exercise that is designed for cardiovascular fitness and exercise that's designed for weight loss," says Dr. Van Itallie. "Thirty minutes of aerobic exercise three times a week will improve your cardiovascular condition. But for significant weight loss, I recommend gradually working up to 2 hours of brisk, purposeful walking every day. For maintenance, you can cut back to about an hour a day."

Dr. Blackburn agrees that, if you're exercising to lose weight, frequency and duration take precedence over intensity. "Instead of a strenuous aerobic regimen three times per week, I'd like to see a more moderate routine—say, walking or bicycling—five to seven days a week," he says. Of course, the more time you can devote to exercise, the better. But to be realistic, he says, most people would do well if they could walk for 40 minutes a day.

HOW TO GET PAST THAT PLATEAU

Suppose you've embarked on a low-calorie diet and shed 25 to 30 pounds as a result. The weight came off pretty fast. But the diet doesn't seem to be working anymore. You've stalled 10 pounds from your weight goal. How do you get past this plateau?

First, say the experts, congratulate yourself. A 30-pound weight loss is worth celebrating. Reward yourself with a vacation—a vacation from weight loss. That's not to say you should binge back the 30 pounds. Rather, ease up to a maintenance plan.

If you've just dropped a fast 30 pounds, chances are you're in a very different metabolic state than you were before dieting, Dr. Van Itallie explains. The challenge now is to stabilize yourself at the new weight. If you're able to do this for a few months, your body should be better prepared to let go of the last 10 pounds.

Dr. Brownell seconds this "vacation" strategy. "Last year I had the opportunity to meet with a large group of individuals who averaged a 100-pound weight loss. I asked them how they overcame their weight-loss plateaus. Several said that they took a break from dieting and maintained their losses for a period of time before they took up dieting again," he explains.

To maintain a lower weight, you can eat more than you did while dieting but less than you ate at the higher weight.

"Keep in mind that for every pound you lose, you will burn 10 calories less per day just because you are lighter," says Dr. Blackburn. "So, to maintain a 30-pound loss, you'll have to eat 300 calories a day less or burn 300 calories a day more than you did at your higher weight."

"You probably have to change the nature of your diet, too, so that you're eating foods lower in fat and higher in complex carbohydrates," Dr. Van Itallie adds, "and adjust your life-style to make more room for exercise."

Only after you've maintained the 30-pound loss for at least three to six months should you tackle the last 10 pounds, a panel of experts agreed. When you're ready, then, follow the advice given for the first scenario: Take it slowly, eat a moderately reduced high-carbohydrate diet, and gear yourself up for an hour or so of brisk walking every day.

Suppose you've repeatedly lost and gained 10 pounds. Now, you're finding it virtually impossible to take them off again. What can you do to put an end to weight cycling and rid yourself of this unwanted weight once and for all?

"If you've lost before, this time you may have a more difficult battle to fight," says Dr. Brownell. "This doesn't mean that you won't lose this weight. But there is a possibility it's going to take more—more calorie cuts, more exercise and most important, more motivation and commitment."

"People who continually regain their losses are obviously on the wrong track," says Dr. Van Itallie. "Those people have to take a careful look at their life-style and see whether, in fact, they are willing to commit themselves to permanent changes.

"Ask yourself: Am I really prepared to walk or bicycle for an hour a day every day for the rest of my life? Am I really prepared to permanently give up fried foods, fatty meats and whole milk in favor of fruits, vegetables, fish and other low-fat, high-fiber fare? If you can't answer yes, without hesitation, to those questions, then it's a waste of time, energy and emotion to lose those 10 pounds. You'll only gain them back—again."

However (here's the best news), if you can answer with a resounding yes, your battle of the bulge is as good as won.

21

101 Little Ways to Lose a Lot of Weight

"Your extra weight is the final result of many small behavioral acts, things like eating between meals or driving to places only two blocks away," explains Kelly Brownell, Ph.D., co-director of the Obesity Research Center at the University of Pennsylvania School of Medicine in Philadelphia. "So you can lose weight by making many small, clever changes—in diet, exercise and attitude."

I agree, Kelly. So here we go.

1. Fidgeting, for those of us who habitually squirm, toe tap or finger drum, has been found in one study to burn up to 800 calories a day in some people. That's the equivalent of jogging several miles. "You really can't make your body have more spontaneous activity like fidgeting if you don't already do it," explains Eric Ravussin, Ph.D., visiting scientist with the National Institutes of Health in Bethesda, Maryland, and one of the study's researchers. "You can, however, decide to make your body work more when-

101 Little Ways to Lose a Lot of Weight

ever possible to burn extra calories. Try doing things like getting up to switch TV channels by hand instead of by remote control," he advises, "or putting frequently used books on higher shelves so you have to reach."

2. Share desserts if skipping them is unthinkable.

3. Downscale your brand of ice cream. If it'll be a cold day in Key West before your freezer doesn't have a carton of this confection waiting for you, buy the least expensive or a reduced-fat brand. Your intake of fat and calories will be considerably lower than if you ate the gourmet kind.

4. Don't eat foods out of their original containers. You may think you're having "just a tad," but you'll probably consume more than if you had dished out the food in a measured portion.

5. Don't bring your "weakness food" into the house. Present yourself with the hassle of going to the store for single servings if you can't fight off a craving. This way you'll either get some exercise (especially if you walk to the store) or you'll decide the snack isn't worth the bother after all.

6. Go grocery shopping on a full stomach. Nacho chips, doughnuts and other tempters won't have half the allure they would if you hunted through those aisles hungry.

7. Shop from a list of necessities. Allow yourself only one purchase that wasn't preplanned.

8. Take only a limited amount of money to the grocery store as an extra reinforcement against buying high-calorie foods.

9. Swear off elevators and escalators. Take the stairs.

10. Police your eating speed by putting your fork down between bites. The more slowly you eat, the more quickly you'll feel full.

11. Establish a time-out routine halfway through your meals. One trick: Put a large pot of water on the stove when you sit down to eat. When it boils (in about 10 or 15 minutes), get up and make a pot of herb tea. When you go back to the table, you probably won't feel like eating much more.

12. Fire the maid and do your own housework. Depending on your body weight, studies show you can burn 195 to

305 calories for each hour you spend washing windows, mopping floors and doing other tasks.

13. Deautomate your housework and make your body work harder. Wash dishes, mix batters and open cans by hand, and hang your wash on the line instead of using a dryer.

14. Use whipped or softened butter or margarine. You'll spread the flavor around using a lot less than if it were hard and you had to scrape it on.

15. Learn that it's okay to say an assertive, "No, thank you" when other people offer you food.

16. Hold a conference and explain your weight-loss wish to family, friends or doughnut-bearing co-workers. Ask them to understand if you turn down their dinners or candy.

17. Go out dancing, miniature golfing, bowling—anything active—if you normally sit around and play bridge or watch television. The most calories you can burn in an hour playing cards is 95, but waltzing can whisk away 195 to 305 for every hour on the floor, and an hour of square dancing can stomp away 330 to 510 calories.

18. Drink no-calorie sparkling waters when you're out, instead of alcoholic beverages.

19. Get rid of those degrading signs and pictures on your refrigerator—no 300-pound women in bikinis or pink pigs on beach blankets to shame you into not eating. Your willpower will be stronger from encouragement, not belittlement.

20. Set a realistic goal for yourself. "Take it one day at a time and don't punish yourself for slipping," says Suzann Johnson, a registered nutritionist with Weight Watchers International. "You'll be more successful if you remember to be your own best friend."

21. Exercise during television commercials. Those 3-minute spurts will keep you out of the kitchen.

22. Use good plate psychology. Don't use place settings with intense colors such as violet, lime green, bright yellow or bright blue; they're thought to stimulate the appetite. The same goes for primitive-looking pewter and wooden plates. Instead, appease your appetite with elegant place settings in darker colors. Choose plates with broad decorative

borders and a slightly "bowled" design. You can fit less food in them.

23. Leave the table as soon as you're finished eating, instead of lingering over the last bites.
24. Eat only at scheduled times in scheduled places.
25. Don't eat everything on your plate (unless you're having steamed vegetables and fish, or an equally good-for-you meal).
26. Have someone else serve you, and ask for smaller portions.
27. Remove food stashed in inappropriate places. Get the candy bars out of your desk drawer and remove the nut bowl from the coffee table.
28. Chew each bite of food at least ten times to really taste it and to make yourself eat more slowly.
29. Don't skip meals. You'll only overeat later.
30. Invite your spouse or housemate into the kitchen with you when you're preparing meals and cleaning up to keep you from sampling as you go.
31. Start your diet with a food diary. Record everything you eat, what you were doing at the time, how you felt. That tells you about yourself—your temptation times, the emotional states that encourage you to nosh—and may help you lose weight, once you see how much you eat.
32. If you're about to cheat, allow yourself a treat, then eat only half and throw the other half away.
33. When hunger hits, wait several minutes before eating and see if it passes.
34. Instead of eating the forbidden piece of candy, brush your teeth. The sweetness of the toothpaste may take your craving away.
35. Drink six to eight glasses of water a day. Water itself helps cut down on water retention because it acts as a diuretic. Taken before meals, it dulls the appetite by giving you that "full" feeling.
36. Diet with a buddy. Many successful weight-loss programs rely heavily on support groups: caring people who help one another succeed. Start your own, even with just one other person.
37. Avoid evening TV. Studies show that people who watch a lot of TV tend to be overweight. Overweight people will

tell you that TV encourages them not only to sit still but also to snack.

38. Substitute activity for eating. When the cravings hit, go to the Y, or dust, or walk around the block. This is especially helpful if you eat out of anger.

39. If you're a late-late-night eater, have a carbohydrate, such as a slice of bread or a cracker, before bedtime to cut down on cravings. Keep an orange slice or a glass of water by your bed to quiet the hunger pangs that wake you up.

40. Go ahead and buy the candy, but don't eat it right away. If you wait, you might decide it's not worth the calories.

41. If you use food as a reward, establish a new reward system. Buy yourself flowers instead of candy.

42. Write down everything you eat—everything, including what you taste when you cook. If you monitor what you eat, you can't go off the diet.

43. If you plateau at a certain weight, don't panic. It's your body getting used to the new you. Drink water, increase your exercise or reduce your calories (don't go below 1,000) to give you the boost you need.

44. Weigh yourself once a week at the same time. Your weight fluctuates constantly and you can weigh more at night than you did in the morning, a downer if you stuck to your diet all day.

45. Feel like you're about to really pig out? Quickly suck on something sour: a pickle or lemon. If you suck it for a while, you may eliminate your cravings.

46. If you want something sweet, eat the smallest amount of fruit or sip the tiniest amount of fruit juice you can to get you through the crisis.

47. If the pie on the counter is just too great a temptation and you don't want to throw it away, freeze it.

48. Make your own sweet drink by adding a little bit of vanilla to ice water with some artificial sweetener.

49. If a binge is about to strike, do your nails. A couple of coats of polish take some time to dry, and by then the danger could pass.

50. Use visualization. Imagine yourself 10 pounds heavier. Then add a few more pounds. Ask yourself if you still

really want to eat. Then close your eyes and imagine yourself at your ideal weight.

51. Make dining an event. Eat from your own special plate, on your own special place mat, and borrow the Japanese art of food arranging to make your meal, however meager, look lovely. This is a trick that helps chronic overeaters and bingers pay attention to their food, instead of consuming it unconsciously.

52. Avoid finger foods that are easy to eat in large amounts.

53. Avoid consuming large quantities of fattening liquids, which are so easy to overdo. That includes alcohol.

54. Keep plenty of crunchy foods like raw veggies and air-popped popcorn on hand. They're high in fiber, and they're satisfying and filling.

55. Eat with a cocktail fork.

56. Don't lose too quickly. Be happy with a slower weight loss. Remember, you're less likely to gain back what you lose slowly and your body isn't going to sag.

57. Don't eat with the radio or stereo on. Concentrate on eating every mouthful slowly and savoring each morsel.

58. Use chopsticks. Unless you're really adept, you'll be forced to eat more slowly and take smaller bites.

59. Always eat with a utensil—even finger foods like fruit or bread.

60. Buy nonstick pans so you can sauté without the addition of any fat.

61. Wear a belt or girdle that makes you aware of when you've eaten enough.

62. When eating out, eat your salad first, with low-calorie dressing or lemon, to dull your appetite before the entree.

63. Lose weight for yourself, not for your husband, your mother or your friends.

64. Make the kitchen off-limits at any time other than mealtime.

65. Blaze walking trails away from tempting sweet shops or hot-dog vendors.

66. Use smaller plates than usual.

67. Get enough sleep—but not too much.

68. Try to avoid sugar. It tends to make you crave more and more.

69. Lose 2 pounds more than your ideal weight to give you some leeway when your weight fluctuates.
70. Plan ahead. Know what you're going to have to eat tomorrow and schedule leftovers into your meal plans. A weekly meal planner is ideal.
71. Switch your late-night snacks to early breakfasts. Studies have shown that people who eat 2,000 calories in the morning lose more weight than those who eat the same amount at night.
72. When eating out, order your food first, then your drinks. This will probably cut down on the amount of drinks you'll have time for.
73. Say "adios" to the pīna colada. Serving for serving, this cocktail is the most caloric alcoholic drink in the known universe, tipping the scales at up to 450 calories or more each.
74. Dilute fruit juices and alcoholic beverages with water or sparkling soda.
75. If you sample all the way through a meal preparation and you're full when it's time to sit down to eat, admit it! Arrange your dinner on a plate, cover with aluminum foil and freeze for a future "TV" dinner.
76. Read or listen to other people's weight-loss success stories and avoid people who are stuck on excuses. Nothing is more inspirational and motivating than knowing that others have been able to do what you wish to accomplish.
77. Freeze fresh fruit, like grapes or strawberries. They'll take longer to eat and you'll be satisfied with less.
78. Leave sugar-hungry kids at home when you go grocery shopping. If you've got a sweet tooth, Junior's extra coaxing may push you over the edge toward that box of chocolate chip cookies or devil's food cake.
79. Plan definite nonfood rewards for yourself as you drop pounds and for other accomplishments in your life. If you get a raise, celebrate by doing something you've always wanted to do but couldn't afford, like a hot-air balloon ride, instead of blowing 100 bucks on a fancy dinner.
80. Learn to love MTV. If you must be at home in front of the TV, take half-hour dance breaks. Feel your body move and forget that it's exercise.

81. Walk the dog instead of letting him out the back door or chaining him up. You'll both be happier and healthier for doing this.
82. Sip soup. A hot bowl of low-calorie soup can be wonderfully filling. Serve as an appetizer to cut down calorie consumption at dinner, or plan a meal with a high-fiber salad to complement it.
83. Substitute plain yogurt for mayonnaise and sour cream in dips and dressings and on baked potatoes.
84. Boost your sagging energy with a brisk walk rather than a sweet snack. Studies show not only that a 10-minute stroll will give you more energy but also that the energy will last longer and you'll feel less tense.
85. Learn to make simple foods seductive. There's more to a meal than meets the stomach. Eating a radish that's been carved into a rose can be a sensual experience. Pastry isn't the only food that can be beautiful.
86. If you're trying to quit smoking and lose weight, see your doctor about a prescription for nicotine gum. Nicotine apparently speeds metabolism and suppresses appetite, and the gum may help cap weight gain in those first months of withdrawal.
87. Plan a walking vacation at least three months in advance and start preparing for it by walking a few miles every day. Get a travel poster of your destination and pin it to your refrigerator. Imagine yourself wearing shorts on the trip.
88. Avoid boredom. There is probably no bigger diet buster. Too often, time on your hands translates to food in your mouth. Know when you'll have big stretches of free time and plan an enjoyable activity. If your plan is to do some much-needed daydreaming, do it far from any food source.
89. Know your fast food. The difference between a three-piece Kentucky Fried Chicken dinner and a McDonald's hamburger is 660 calories. Proceed with caution when you pull up to any drive-in window.
90. Vary your exercise routine to avoid boredom. And take it easy. Researchers at Kings College in England found that women who tried strenuous exercise couldn't do it long enough or hard enough to burn many calories.

91. Use your mirror to judge your progress. It's more reliable than the fluctuating number of pounds you weigh. Sometimes you may weigh more but your clothes will fit better due to toning and muscle development from exercising.

92. Bulk up—with muscle, not fat. Muscle burns more calories than fat, so exercise that builds muscles is working for you double time by burning calories as well as creating muscles that burn even more calories.

93. Chew sugarless gum for oral gratification or to keep your mouth occupied when you're preparing food. It may be helpful in ending a meal, too.

94. Invest in a hot-air popcorn popper. Enjoy snacks of oil-free popcorn. No muss, no fuss and lots fewer calories than conventionally popped stuff.

95. Think of meat as a condiment to vegetables, grains or pasta. Buy smaller quantities and cut up to add to fiber-rich main dishes.

96. Eat a midmorning snack if an early morning breakfast is too tough. It will help curb your midafternoon cravings.

97. Give away the "fat" clothes in your closet. Keeping larger sizes around undermines your confidence in being able to maintain your weight loss.

98. If you must buy fattening foods for nondieters in your family, buy varieties you don't like. If you're hopelessly addicted to chocolate ice cream, buy your kids strawberry.

99. Sit up straight! Proper posture burns more calories than slouching, and besides, it makes your belly look better.

100. Choose whole wheat matzo or Scandinavian imports when shopping for crackers to munch on. They have the lowest calories per ounce and no fat.

101. Turn down the stereo. Noise can be fattening! Loud noise produces stress chemicals that may make people overeat.

MY OWN "LITTLE WAYS" TO LOSE WEIGHT

Fill in this space with an idea of your own once a week. And each time you do that, study what you have written before. Doing so will help you maintain a high consciousness of your eating behavior, the key to successful, permanent weight loss.

Height and Weight and Body Frame Tables

The first of the following tables gives the range of desirable weights for men and women of various heights. It was developed by the Metropolitan Life Insurance Companies, based on the weights and life expectancy of some of their policyholders. Generally speaking, people whose weights fall within these ranges have a smaller risk of premature death than those who weigh more (or less) than the given weights. While this table can't tell you exactly to the pound how much you should weigh—or whether or not weighing slightly more poses any kind of health risk—the weight ranges can help you set a goal for your individual ideal weight.

Note that the heights listed assume that men are wearing 1-inch heels and women 2-inch heels. If you know your height in bare feet, add the appropriate number of inches to find your height in the table. If you usually weigh yourself without clothing, subtract 5 pounds if you are a man and 3 pounds if you are a woman.

Body frame (which is based on bone structure, not overall mass) also figures into your desirable weight. The second table below provides a method to quickly and easily determine whether you are small-, medium- or large-framed.

DESIRABLE WEIGHTS FOR ADULTS
(AGE 25 AND OVER)

Height (in shoes*)	Weight in Lbs. (in indoor clothing)		
	Small Frame	Medium Frame	Large Frame
Men			
5' 2"	112–120	118–129	126–141
5' 3"	115–123	121–133	129–144
5' 4"	118–126	124–136	132–148
5' 5"	121–129	127–139	135–152
5' 6"	124–133	130–143	138–156
5' 7"	128–137	134–147	142–161
5' 8"	132–141	138–152	147–166
5' 9"	136–145	142–156	151–170
5'10"	140–150	146–160	155–174
5'11"	144–154	150–165	159–179
6' 0"	148–158	154–170	164–184
6' 1"	152–162	158–175	168–189
6' 2"	156–167	162–180	173–194
6' 3"	160–171	167–185	178–199
6' 4"	164–175	172–190	182–204
Women			
4'10"	92– 98	96–107	104–119
4'11"	94–101	98–110	106–122
5' 0"	96–104	101–113	109–125
5' 1"	99–107	104–116	112–128
5' 2"	102–110	107–119	115–131
5' 3"	105–113	110–122	118–134
5' 4"	108–116	113–126	121–138
5' 5"	111–119	116–130	125–142
5' 6"	114–123	120–135	129–146
5' 7"	118–127	124–139	133–150
5' 8"	122–131	128–143	137–154
5' 9"	126–135	132–147	141–158
5'10"	130–140	136–151	145–163
5'11"	134–144	140–155	149–168
6' 0"	138–148	144–159	153–173

SOURCE: Adapted from *Statistical Bulletin,* Vol. 58 (New York: Metropolitan Life Insurance Company, October 1977). Based on Build and Blood Pressure Study, 1959, Society of Actuaries.
*1-inch heels for men and 2-inch heels for women.

DETERMINING YOUR BODY FRAME

Extend your arm and bend your forearm upward at a 90-degree angle. Keep your fingers straight and turn the inside of your wrist away from your body. Place the thumb and index finger of your other hand on the two prominent bones on *either side* of your elbow. Measure the space between your fingers against a ruler or a tape measure. (For the most accurate measurement, you can have your physician measure your elbow breadth with a caliper.) Compare the measurements on the following tables.

This table lists the elbow measurements for medium-framed men and women of various heights. Measurements lower than those listed indicate you have a small frame, and higher measurements indicate a large frame.

Height in 1-in. Heels	Elbow Breadth (in.)
Men	
5' 2"–5' 3"	2½–2⅞
5' 4"–5' 7"	2⅝–2⅞
5' 8"–5'11"	2¾–3
6' 0"–6' 3"	2¾–3⅛
6' 4"	2⅞–3¼
Women	
4'10"–4'11"	2¼–2½
5' 0"–5' 3"	2¼–2½
5' 4"–5' 7"	2⅜–2⅝
5' 8"–5'11"	2⅜–2⅝
6' 0"	2½–2¾

SOURCE: Metropolitan Life Insurance Company, 1983.

B

How Many Calories Do You Need?

To keep your weight steady, you must take in the same number of calories that you burn. But just exactly how do you determine what that number is? Choose the life-style below that's closest to yours, plug your weight into the simple formula and multiply by the number given. The answer is your daily calorie need. To lose weight, of course, either cut the calories or exercise more.

Extremely inactive. You have a job that keeps you at a desk virtually all day. You never exercise. Your motto is, "Why walk when I can ride?" You like sports—on TV.

$$\underline{\hspace{2cm}} \times 13 = \underline{\hspace{2cm}}$$

Less active than average. You are sedentary on your job. Less than once a week you bestir yourself for a small amount of exercise. You don't like walking. The elevator is your good friend.

$$\underline{\hspace{2cm}} \times 14 = \underline{\hspace{2cm}}$$

231

Reasonably active. You take part in an active sport once or twice a week. You also walk. Or your job requires you to exert yourself for at least 15 minutes each day.

_____ × 15 = _____

Very active. At least three times a week, you perform vigorous exercise like running, swimming or handball for an hour. You walk and use stairs. Or hard physical labor fills 40 percent of your workday.

_____ × 17 = _____

Extremely active. You may be an athlete in training. You run 10 miles a day or perform an equivalent activity. Or your job demands heavy physical exertion from you 70 percent of the time.

_____ × 21 = _____

C

Calorie Counts of Various Activities

If you enjoy paying compulsive attention to numbers, you are better off lavishing your energy on the calories burned by exercise than on the calories contained in food. You can only manipulate your diet so much, cut back so many calories, before you begin to feel deprived and genuinely hungry. But if you manipulate your daily schedule to permit an extra hour of easy walking, you can burn, for instance, another 300 calories a day without having to worry about physical or psychological backlash. Sure, the first few days your legs will be a little sore, but after a week or so, there will be no strain if you are in normal health.

The table in this appendix is also useful in assessing, in approximate terms, the caloric costs of your daily routine. It's especially useful, I think, in pinpointing the effect of changing habits. Let's assume, for instance, that you are a 48-year-old woman and that you are now considerably heavier than you were 25 years ago, even though you're convinced you're eating less than you used to. But perhaps as the years passed, you changed your routine in a number of seemingly minor ways. Looking at the table, you'll be able to see what effect these changes have had. Back then, you might have gone dancing once a week, which would have burned up about 220 calories. You went bowling once a week, which burned up another 150 calories. On weekends, you waitressed for a total of 12 hours, which consumed 2,280 calories. The kids were home then, so you did a lot more housework, and in those days, you used to hang your wash out on the line, which burns more calories than using a dryer. You estimate the weekly decrease in "housework calories" at 400. Add it all up and your total decrement on a weekly basis—compared to what you expended at age 23—amounts to about 3,050 calories.

Of course, you aren't spending all that additional time sleeping, but instead of hanging out wash, scrubbing floors and bowling, your new activities are more in the line of driving a car, sewing and watching TV. If you add up the additional hours that you now spend in such activities, you might come up with a total of, say, 850. Subtracting that from 3,050 gives you a net weekly exercise decrement equivalent to 2,200 calories, or about 315 a day.

And what do those 315 extra calories a day mean? Quite precisely, they mean about 22 extra pounds of weight. Remember that every extra pound of fat you're carrying causes you to burn up another 14 calories. So to find out at what point your added weight will cause you to stop gaining weight, you would only have to divide 315 by 14, which turns out to be 22.5.

So much for diagnosis. Now let's talk about cure.

Bowling no longer interests you, you say, and you'd need a team of draft horses to pull your husband out to a dance. Nor does scrubbing floors or hanging out your wash especially appeal to you. Well, what about swimming? If you swam at the rate of only 20 yards per minute, which is an extremely slow pace, permitting frequent rests, you could burn up—assuming that you now weigh about 150 pounds—some 150 calories in half an hour. Do that three times a week and you're subtracting a total of 450 calories. What about walking? Three miles an hour is a very comfortable pace, and if you walk for an hour four times a week, that's another 1,200 calories. And let's say that you return to the piano you've forgotten about, and substitute an hour of piano playing every day for an hour of TV watching. That's another 280 calories a week. All of which gives you an additional 2,490 calories a week, enough to produce a weight loss of 20 pounds. If, at the same time, you reduce your daily food intake to the tune of 300 calories a day, the losing won't stop until you have lost 40 pounds, which will take you very nicely back to where you were 25 years ago. But long before you reach that level, you will have gained so much new energy that you'll be walking more, swimming more and probably enjoying many other activities as well, which will speed your weight loss along that much faster.

A word or two about the technical side of this table is now in order. First, the caloric values given include the calories you are burning up as a result of your Basal Metabolic Rate, frequently referred to as the BMR. Those are the calories that you spend on such basic chores as circulating your blood, breathing and digesting your food. The average figure usually given for the BMR is about 50 calories an hour—essentially the same number of calories expended when sleeping, when you aren't doing anything but your BMR act. If you are considerably overweight, your BMR will naturally be higher, but 50 is a useful approximation.

That means that when the table says that if you weigh 150 pounds and walk for an hour at 3 miles per hour, you'll burn up 300 calories, what it really means is that you'll burn up 250 calories more than you would by doing nothing, which burns up 50. That difference would possibly appear to be serious if you use these figures to calculate the additional calories (above normal calorie expenditure) you'll be burning through exercise. In other words, an hour of walking is only burning up an additional 250, instead of 300, calories, calories that you wouldn't expend if you were watching TV. However, these higher values are so commonly used that I have used them myself throughout the book. There is, though, a saving grace that in many cases will make up the difference—and maybe even more—very nicely.

Edward Watt, Ph.D., cardiovascular physiologist at the Preventive Cardiology Clinic in Atlanta, Georgia, says that in calculating the calories burned by exercise, it's important to add the time to return to the preexercise resting rate. Because the increase in metabolic rate can continue for from 30 minutes to several hours after exercise is discontinued, the number of calories consumed by the exercise is significantly greater than this table indicates.

That was quite a revelation to me, and it explains why vigorous exercise seems to produce weight loss beyond what you'd expect, while very light exercise, like ironing, which does not really raise your metabolic rate, seems disproportionately small in its effect. Moral: To the extent that your exercise gets you sweating, it's giving you a calorie-loss bonus by burning fuel even after you've showered.

CALORIE COSTS PER HOUR
OF SOME COMMON DAILY ACTIVITIES

Activity	Weight (lb.)		
	110–125	150	180–200
Assembly line work			
Light	150–175	220	260
Medium	205	260	305
Heavy	230	295	340
Bricklaying	160	205	235
Calisthenics	235	300	350
Carpentry			
Light	150–180	175–230	200–270
Heavy	280	355	415
Chopping wood			
By hand	355	400–450	525
Using power saw	175	220	260
Stacking wood	300	380	400–440

Calorie Counts of Various Activities

Be aware also that the values given here are, quite naturally, approximate, and they depend largely on the degree of vigor with which the given activity is pursued. Also, if you do not pursue a given activity for one solid hour, simply divide by two for half an hour, three for 20 minutes and so forth.

Equivalent Activities and Remarks

1 hr. light carpentry or making beds.
1 hr. scrubbing floors or waitressing.
¾ hr. bicycling at 10 mph, hiking at 2 mph with 20-lb. pack or playing tennis (doubles); 1 hr. walking at 3 mph.

½ hr. chopping wood by hand or 1 hr. cutting wood with power saw; 1 hr. painting house; 2 hr. typing.

1 hr. hiking at 2 mph with 20-lb. pack; ½ hr. playing handball; 1 hr. swimming at easy pace. For optimum fitness, calisthenics should be combined to use muscles of the whole body in order to be as valuable as swimming, tennis handball, etc. Begin with relaxation and limbering routine to warm up; after workout, use relaxation techniques again. Main disadvantage is that calisthenics can be boring unless done in groups or to music.

1 hr. washing and polishing car; 1 hr. driving truck; 20 min. playing handball; 35 min. walking at 4 mph.
1 hr. playing volleyball; 1 hr. walking at 4 mph.

2 hr. cutting wood with power saw.
½ hr. chopping wood by hand; 25 min. playing handball.
1 hr. gardening; 1 hr. playing golf, carrying clubs.

(continued)

CALORIE COSTS PER HOUR
OF SOME COMMON DAILY ACTIVITIES—*Continued*

	Weight (lb.)		
Activity	110–125	150	180–200
Dancing			
In general	240–250	270	300–450
Light	215	275	320
Rock	195	250	295
Square	330	350–420	480
Domestic work			
Baking	107	137	162
Cleaning windows	180–195	210–250	295
Ironing	160	205	235–240
Making beds	165–200	210–240	245–300
Preparing dinner	105	135	155
Scrubbing floors	195	250	295
Sewing, knitting	75	95	110
Shopping	130–150	165	195–200
Washing and drying clothes			
Using washing machine	125–150	160	190
Using dryer	125–150	160	190
Hanging on line	190	245	285–300
Washing dishes			
By hand	105	135	155
Using dishwasher	60–85	110	130

Calorie Counts of Various Activities

Equivalent Activities and Remarks

1 hr. gardening; ¾ hr. bicycling at 10 mph. Calorie expenditure for dancing usually falls in the range of 270 to 460 and is governed by tempo of the music as well as individual style and enthusiasm.

35 min. easy cycling; 15 min. skipping rope. Values are less if using a mixer, more if beating batter by hand. Many recipes require both.

1 hr. hanging clothes on line; 25 min. skipping rope; 3 hr. watching TV.

2½ hr. watching TV; 50 min. waitressing. Ironing burns up considerably more calories than just standing, due to lifting and pushing the weight of the iron and hanging pressed clothes.

1 hr., 10 min. walking at 2 mph; 1 hr. practicing yoga; 1 hr. washing and polishing car; ¾ hr. swimming or calisthenics.

Basically the same as for standing only, unless you are whipping eggs, flipping a pizza shell, bending and opening drawers, etc.

Scrubbing floors *can* burn up to 420 calories per hr.

About the same as reading. Both slightly more than just sitting and watching TV.

This is light shopping. Carrying heavy packages will increase calorie loss by 100.

Modern equipment makes household tasks easier today, but it may not seem that way if you are not physically fit.

(continued)

CALORIE COSTS PER HOUR
OF SOME COMMON DAILY ACTIVITIES—*Continued*

Activity	Weight (lb.)		
	110–125	150	180–200
Dressing, undressing, washing, showering, brushing hair	150–160	205	235
Driving car			
Light traffic	60–75	95–100	100–115
Heavy traffic	80–105	100–135	155–180
Driving truck (tractor-trailer)	180	230	270
Gardening			
Weeding, hoeing, digging, spading	240–305	300–390	400–450
Raking	175	220	260
Mowing lawn			
Pushing power mower	210	270	310
Using riding mower	115	145	170
Painting house	165	210	245
Playing piano	95	120	145
Reading	70	90	105

Calorie Counts of Various Activities

Equivalent Activities and Remarks

In most cases, 1 hr. per day is taken up by these activities.

Higher values are for standard vs. automatic transmissions.

1 hr. washing and polishing car; 1 hr. raking; 20 min. light snow shoveling; 50 min. easy rowing.

Attitude and zeal will dictate variations in calories lost here. 220 to 300 calories/hr. is a good rule of thumb, if you are hoeing beans or pampering azaleas.

¾ hr. playing tennis (doubles) or hiking at 2 mph with 20-lb. pack; 22 min. playing handball or light snow shoveling.

Pushing your mower instead of sitting on it will burn up almost twice as many calories.

1 hr. cleaning windows, light assembly line work, or light carpentry; ¾ hr. playing tennis (doubles); 2¾ hr. watching TV.

A lively piece such as Liszt's "Tarantella" requires one-third more energy than Beethoven's "Appassionata" and two and a half times as much as Mendelssohn's songs.

Burns same amount of calories as writing, slightly more than just sitting or watching TV, and less than typing.

(continued)

CALORIE COSTS PER HOUR
OF SOME COMMON DAILY ACTIVITIES—*Continued*

	Weight (lb.)		
Activity	110–125	150	180–200
Running			
5½ mph (easy jogging)	515	655	760
8 mph	625	800	930
11 mph	955	1,220	1,420
12½ mph (very fast)	1,200	1,550	1,805
Sex			
Foreplay	80	100	115
Intercourse			
Vigorous	235	300	350
Easy	105	135	155
Shoveling snow (light)	475	610	710
Sitting	60	80	90
Skipping rope (75 skips/min.)	435	555	645
Sleeping	50	65–80	80
Sports			
Bicycling (geared bike, average terrain)			
5 mph (easy)	190	245	280
10–12 mph (moderate)	240–325	270–415	300–475
13–15 mph (vigorous)	515	660–720	760
Bowling	150	190	240

Calorie Counts of Various Activities

Equivalent Activities and Remarks

How far you run is more important than how fast you run. Unfit people should design a stretching and calisthenics program for themselves before taking up running in order to avoid knee pain, back pain or muscle strains.

Burns slightly fewer calories than typing.

Same as hiking or swimming for the vigorous approach or playing piano for the easy approach.

1 hr. playing handball; 2 hr. walking at 3 mph; playing tennis (doubles); or swimming at 20 mph or 20 yd./min.

1 hr. watching TV; 6 min. playing handball; 20 min. light assembly line work or carpentry; 15 min. gardening; 13 min. walking at 4 mph.

1½ hr. walking at 4 mph or playing volleyball; 7 hr. watching TV. Do this as a "coffee break" to get your energy up and to avoid the doughnuts and Danish. Running shoes are advisable to avoid ankle and knee damage.

Also equivalent to lying awake in bed. Does not vary much from Basal Metabolism Rate.

Energy cost of sports are approximate, influenced by the vigor of the individual participant.

If you cycle 6 miles to and from work instead of driving, taking about 30 min. each way, you could burn 15 to 20 lb. of fat a year.

This is regular bowling rather than continuous bowling. Possibility of taking in more calories in food and beverages than are burned up makes bowling a doubtful weight-loss activity.

(continued)

CALORIE COSTS PER HOUR
OF SOME COMMON DAILY ACTIVITIES—*Continued*

	Weight (lb.)		
Activity	110–125	150	180–200
Sports—*continued*			
Fishing			
From boat	105	135	155
Wading	235	300	350
Golf			
Twosome, carrying clubs	295	380	440
Twosome, pulling clubs	260	335	385
Foursome, carrying clubs	210	270	310
Foursome, pulling clubs	195	250	295
Handball	470	600	695
Hiking, 2 mph (20-lb. pack)	235	300	350
Hill climbing	470	600	695
Riding horseback			
Walking	130	165	195
Trotting	325	415	475
Rowing			
Easy	235	300	350
Vigorous	515	655	760
Skiing			
Downhill, excluding lifts	465	595	690
Cross-country, 5 mph	550	700	800

Equivalent Activities and Remarks

40 min. slow walking; 25 min. swimming or calisthenics.
½ hr. hill climbing; 1 hr. calisthenics.

Not much better than walking unless you carry your clubs, play on a hilly course or jog around the course before each round. If you use a caddy or electric cart, forget it!

2 hr. walking at 3 mph; 55 min. vigorous rowing or moderate swimming; 8 hr. watching TV. A vigorous workout provides a maximum of exercise in a minimum of time. Remember to warm up first.
4 hr. watching TV; ¾ hr. gardening; 1¼ hr. washing and polishing car; 1 hr. walking at 3 mph; 22 min. running at 8 mph; ½ hr. playing handball; 40 min. playing table tennis.
1 hr. playing handball; 55 min. moderate swimming; 3 hr. bowling; 1 hr. downhill skiing, excluding lifts; 1¾ hr. brisk walking.

1 hr. light shopping; 50 min. bowling or slow walking.
1 hr. square dancing; ½ hr. running at 8 mph.

Easy rowing is equal to 1 hr. hiking at 2 mph with 20-lb. pack or swimming at 20 yd./min. Vigorous rowing is equal to 1 hr. 8 min. playing handball, 1 hr. running at 5½ mph or 1 hr. swimming at 45 yd./min. You will burn more calories in choppy water on a windy day.

Calorie cost is maximized by low temperatures. Excellent activity for fitness and endurance because skiing uses all major muscle groups. The amount of uphill skiing required by cross-country terrain will influence the number of calories burned.

(continued)

CALORIE COSTS PER HOUR
OF SOME COMMON DAILY ACTIVITIES—*Continued*

Activity	Weight (lb.) 110–125	150	180–200
Sports—*continued*			
Swimming			
20 yd./min.	235	300	350
35 yd./min.	425	540	630
55 yd./min.	660	835	975
Table tennis	355	360–450	525
Tennis (recreational)			
Singles	335	425	495
Doubles	235	300	350
Volleyball (recreational)	275	350	405
Wrestling	620	790	920
Standing	105	135–140	155
Typing	80–90	105–115	120–135
Waitressing	190	245	285
Walking			
2 mph	145	185	215
3 mph	235	300	350
4 mph	270	345	405

Equivalent Activities and Remarks

Also uses practically all the muscle groups of the body. Should be balanced by some weight-bearing exercise such as running for all-around muscular development. If you cannot gauge your swimming speed, you can count on burning from 200 to 700 calories/hr. The butterfly stroke burns up the most calories; the crawl the least.

¾ hr. playing handball; 6 hr. watching TV; 1½ hr. hiking at 2 mph with 20-lb. pack; 33 min. running at 8 mph.

Singles: 1 hr., 25 min. swimming at 20 yd./min.; 33 min. running at 8 mph.

Doubles: 1 hr. swimming at 20 yd./min.; 22 min. running at 8 mph.

Depends on how you play the game: If you run for every ball, you will burn more calories than an opponent who considers it a waste of time to run for a shot that will put him out of position.

1 hr. walking at 4 mph; 40 min. skipping rope; 1 hr., 10 min. calisthenics; ¾ hr. chopping wood by hand.

Slightly less than vigorous swimming.

35 min. walking at 2 mph.

1 hr. washing and polishing car.

Calories burned by walking depend on type of surface (asphalt, grass, level, incline), type of clothing and wind resistance, as well as body weight. At approximately 3 mph, you burn 15% more calories walking on grass than on asphalt. Walking up a 15% grade burns up twice as many calories as walking on a level surface. Walking downstairs uses only one-third the calories of walking upstairs. Running upstairs demands even more calories. Climbing upstairs with a load, such as a basket of laundry, burns 11 times as many calories as walking on a level surface carrying the same load.

(continued)

CALORIE COSTS PER HOUR
OF SOME COMMON DAILY ACTIVITIES—*Continued*

Activity	Weight (lb.)		
	110–125	150	180–200
Washing and polishing car	180	230	270
Watching TV	60	80	90
Writing	70	90	105
Yoga	180	230	270

SOURCES: Adapted from
Activetics, by Charles T. Kuntzleman (New York: Peter H. Wyden, 1975).
The Exerciser's Handbook, by Charles T. Kuntzleman (New York: David McKay, 1978).
Frontiers of Fitness, by Roy J. Shepard (Springfield: Charles C. Thomas, 1971).
How Different Sports Rate in Promoting Physical Fitness, by C. Carson Conrad (Washington, D.C.: President's Council on Physical Fitness and Sports, 1978).

Calorie Counts of Various Activities

Equivalent Activities and Remarks

¾ hr. walking at 3 mph; 15 min. running at 8 mph; 25 min. skipping rope; 1 hr. raking; 25 min. playing handball.

40 min. playing piano. The only activity that uses fewer calories is lying in bed and staring at the ceiling.

Same as reading, slightly more than sitting or watching TV, and less than typing.

Value is due to benefits of flexibility and relaxation. Recommended as part of a warm-up routine for more vigorous activities such as running or bicycling.

Human Nutrition, 3d ed., by Benjamin T. Burton (New York: McGraw-Hill, 1976).
Introductory Nutrition, 3d ed., by Helen Andrews Guthrie (St. Louis: C. V. Mosby, 1975).
Textbook of Work Physiology, by Per-Olof Astrand and Kaare Rodahl (New York: McGraw-Hill, 1977).
"Weight Control and Metabolism," by Nigel Oakley, in *Cycling: The Healthy Alternative* (London: British Cycling Bureau, 1978).

APPENDIX

D

Food Rating and Evaluation Guide

The main body of this book has been devoted to teaching you to become more conscious of when and why you are eating. The table in this appendix is devoted to raising your consciousness of *what* you are eating.

By now you already know that it is very unrealistic to choose your diet solely on the basis of its calorie content. On the other hand, it can be *helpful* to know more about the calorie content and nutritional value of various foods and dishes. Using this knowledge as an information resource, rather than as a strict guideline, you'll be able to make better-informed decisions when it comes to choosing among foods you actually like.

There are a number of unusual features in this table, along with the more familiar information, so some brief explanations are in order.

The arithmetic data are taken almost entirely from various publications of the U.S. Department of Agriculture, while in a few cases, values have been obtained from some other sources, such as labels.

However, don't be too impressed with the precise accuracy of these figures, even though most of them are "official." What most people don't realize is that for the most part, the values given in government food tables are "representative," not absolute. The vitamin content of an apple, for instance, will vary somewhat depending on the variety, the weather during the growing season, where the apple was grown, when it was picked and how long it was in shipment and storage before consumption. Government researchers evaluate data from numerous tests and come up with one convenient value. When foods are cooked, even more variables are operating, including the method of cooking, the maximum temperature reached, the length of cooking and how quickly the food was consumed after preparation was completed. Small differences, then, between different foods in this table should not be given much importance, because in reality they are likely to be factitious.

Government researchers, I might also add, use teaspoons that are slightly smaller than most other teaspoons, with the result that the caloric value of a teaspoon of sugar, for example, is given here at 15, while in other tables you may have seen, the figure is 16 or even 18. Such differences are not really important, and I only mention them in the event that you begin comparing data and discover that the values for identical amounts of the same food seem to vary slightly from table to table. You may also be slightly confused if you attempt to find some of the data presented here in government tables, because in certain instances I have done my own calculations to present values for realistic serving sizes.

N/C rating. This is the abbreviation for what I call the Nutrient Value-Caloric Density Ratio. I developed this ratio as a means of expressing the fact that it isn't simply the number of calories that you should worry about, but what you are *getting* for those calories in the way of real nourishment. A bowl of chili con carne, for example, has a lot more calories than an apple, but you will notice that while I give an apple an N/C rating of only "Fair," chili con carne is rated as "Excellent." That's because the greater number of calories in the chili con carne more than pay their way by providing tremendously greater nutritional value.

Likewise, the banana is rated as "Good" while a cup of lima beans (usually considered a no-no to dieters) is rated "Excellent." While a cup of lima beans has almost twice the calories of the banana, it also has ten times as much protein, eight times as much calcium and five times as much iron. The lima beans are also going to be more filling than the banana, which is another factor I tried to take into account in coming up with these ratings.

Keep in mind that these ratings are focused on the needs of the dieter, which may be somewhat different from someone else's needs. The apple we talked about before contains a goodly amount of pectin, which is helpful for someone trying to lower his cholesterol, but the pectin value is not considered in determining the N/C rating. However, the bulk and crunchiness of the apple *were* considered because, while not exactly giving greater nourishment to the apple, they nevertheless make it more desirable to the person who wants to give his mouth and stomach that satisfied feeling.

It hardly needs to be said that N/C ratings can be somewhat debatable. Although I tried to be as objective as possible, I'm certain that many of these ratings could still be justifiably criticized. In certain cases, I may have gone a bit overboard in one direction or another when the food involved enjoys a popular reputation that I don't think is particularly deserved. I doubt that many dietitians would rate apple juice "Poor," as I have done, but so many people abuse this beverage that I think anyone who regularly stocks it in the refrigerator needs to be shaken into realizing that it is far from being a health food.

Protein.   Protein is to your body what wood is to a cottage, what concrete is to a skyscraper and steel is to a bridge. It is the most fundamental building material and plays a critical role in the structure of every tissue and organ of the human anatomy. Even your bones, composed mostly of minerals, require substantial amounts of protein to get all those minerals to hang together.

It is sometimes said that getting enough protein is no problem for Americans, but like so many other things said about the diet of the "average American," that statement can be dangerously misleading. And if you are a relatively small person watching your weight, you would do well to watch your protein intake also. In order to get enough protein to maintain your body in good repair (various parts are always being discarded and replaced), it is advisable for a woman to get between 40 and 60 grams and a man between 50 and 70 daily.

The question is, what do you have to eat to get this amount? It might be instructive to glance at the table for a moment, and add up all the protein provided by typical servings of the first 15 items. In doing so, you'll discover that the total amount of protein contained in a large handful of almonds, a cup of chopped amaranth leaves, an ounce of amaranth grains, one apple, one glass of apple juice, one serving of applesauce, three raw apricots, a serving of dried apricots, a glass of apricot nectar, a serving of asparagus, half an avocado, two slices of bacon, one banana, a cup of green beans and a whole cup of cooked lima beans amounts to a grand total of only 37 grams of protein—not enough for most people's daily requirement.

True, those items aren't exactly a typical daily diet, but there are people who, in an attempt to lose weight quickly, eat almost nothing but fruits, vegetables and grains. That in itself is not bad, providing these vegetable-source foods contain enough protein—protein that is properly balanced. In practice, that means if you are getting your protein from vegetable sources, you should always eat some grain products at the same meal in which you consume legumes such as beans, peas, limas or garbanzos. Or consume nuts along with grain products. Otherwise, you will not get an efficient mixture of amino acids, the components of protein.

Just scanning the table, you will quickly see that a single serving of various kinds of meats or fish will give you more protein than all those other foods we mentioned put together. Eggs, cheese and other dairy products are also rich in protein. Since virtually all lean meats, poultry and fish are given very high ratings in the table, it does make a certain amount of sense to try to include one serving of them in your daily diet—unless, of course, you are a vegetarian. While in some instances a vegetarian will have to consume more calories to get high-quality protein than the person eating lean meat or fish, the vegetarian has the advantage that his sources of protein will probably be a lot more filling. There are also indications that calories are less efficiently absorbed from fiber-rich vegetable foods than from animal foods. On the other hand, the vegetarian who eats large amounts of cheese, peanut butter, oil, ice cream and honey isn't doing his waist a favor. Those foods contain no fiber but lots of calories.

There is another fact about protein which is especially important to the reducer. Many people assume that when you eat slightly less food than you need to maintain your weight, everything you lose is fat. But that is not the case. A substantial but variable amount of the weight lost is actually protein. During fasting, the amount of lean tissue lost may run higher than 50 percent, and this tendency to lose lean tissue instead of fat seems to be particularly strong in older people. (In contrast, when weight is lost as a result of exercise, almost all of that loss is in the form of fat.)

If you follow the reducing approach outlined in this book, which involves eating only 300 or 400 calories a day less than you normally eat, the tendency to lose protein will be minimized. Experience, though, tells me that some people are going to overdo this somewhat, and thus will be losing more protein. In any case, I think it is a good idea for any person on a reducing diet to try to eat 10 to 20 grams more protein than is theoretically required. In other words, I think a woman ought to aim for 50 or 60 grams of protein rather than 40, and a man for 60 or 70 rather than 50.

What happens if you don't get enough protein? Probably the most important things that happen occur at the cellular level, and you may not notice them at all until you have an injury and discover that it's taking an unusually long time to heal. The kind of things you *do* notice may be poor growth of hair; loss of skin tone, producing a haggard look; and perhaps a general sense that you are losing your strength. When you are losing fat, the appearance of your face will change, but it will look younger. If you are losing protein, you will tend to look older, like a person who has just come out of the hospital after a long period of convalescence, which usually causes people to lose very large amounts of protein.

Protein supplements, in my opinion, are necessary only when you are fasting under the supervision of a doctor, or in cases where eating normal foods is very difficult. Chicken, turkey, fish and lean meat have more protein per mouthful than protein tablets, and the protein they deliver is of the very highest quality, whereas some protein supplements are of marginal value. In addition, these natural foods contain important vitamins and minerals lacking in protein supplements. Brewer's yeast or primary (food) yeast are protein supplements I *would* recommend because they are really foods rather than supplements, and they contain generous amounts of vitamins, trace elements and other valuable substances, such as Glucose Tolerance Factor, found in brewer's yeast.

At this point, I should say something about the adjectives such as "excellent" or "scant" which I have appended not only to many protein values in the table but to vitamins and minerals as well. I have done that because I feel that the average person, in scanning a food value table, doesn't really know whether 3 grams of protein, for instance, is a lot or a little, or whether 600 international units of vitamin A is good, bad or indifferent. What I've tried to do is scatter a number of these adjectives throughout the table so that in a few minutes you can easily establish some perspective in judging the significance of the values given. Like the N/C ratings, these adjectives are open to debate, but if nothing else, they are useful guides.

I tend to give higher adjective ratings to vegetable foods that contain useful amounts of protein, since these foods are not ordinarily thought of as protein sources. And there is a growing amount of evidence suggesting that protein from vegetable sources is useful in keeping blood fats down, which protects the circulatory system. I've said it before, but it bears repeating here: Starchy foods like potatoes, corn and beans are *not* fattening.

Calcium. Several people who have lost large amounts of weight—50 pounds or more—on severely restricted diets have told me that they developed chronic backaches after several months of dieting. A major reason for this is almost certainly a lack of sufficient calcium, although insufficient protein could make matters worse. Many adults drink little milk to begin with, and when going on severe diets, they often sharply reduce all dairy products except, perhaps, small amounts of cottage cheese or yogurt. Beef, chicken and fish contain extremely small amounts of calcium—at least in their flesh. Most salad greens and fruits also contain only very small amounts of calcium, and some of the calcium in greens may be difficult for your body to absorb. A number of vegetables contain useful amounts of calcium, but it's unlikely that you'll eat enough of them to meet your requirements. Nutritional researchers have recently suggested that daily calcium intake should be approximately 1,200 to 1,500 milligrams, which is half again as much as, or more than, "official" nutrition tables suggest.

The person most likely to develop a calcium deficiency is a woman past the age of 50 (after menopause, the change in hormones leads to an accelerated loss of calcium from the bones). And if that woman is dieting, or has a history of dieting, the chances of developing a calcium deficiency are extremely high. Symptoms of calcium deficiency may include aches in the middle of the back (low back pain can also be a deficiency symptom), muscle cramping and spasms, and general irritability and nervousness. The slow loss of bone density that occurs during calcium deficiency often has no symptoms at all until, at a relatively advanced age, a fall or even a slight bump that would have been of no consequence 20 years before results in a broken hip. Osteoporosis—the medical name for the loss of bone density—can't even be detected with X-rays until one-third or more of the bone mass has already been lost.

Because calcium is relatively difficult to get in your daily diet, as mentioned before, I recommend that adults—particularly women—take calcium supplements to ensure that they are getting somewhere between 1,000 and 2,000 milligrams of this mineral every day. Still, it pays to make an effort to get calcium from your foods, too, and it's interesting that certain low-calorie foods such as broccoli offer generous amounts of this important mineral.

Iron. If the woman over 50 who is dieting incautiously is likely to develop a calcium deficiency, the woman *under* 50 is more likely to develop an iron deficiency. It is the iron in hemoglobin which carries oxygen throughout the body, and the monthly loss of blood a woman experiences can create serious problems. Iron deficiency can have many symptoms, but the classic deficiency is a sense of profound fatigue. Itching, skin problems, dry hair, dizziness and other conditions you would ordinarily never associate with iron deficiency can also be produced—probably because a reduced flow of oxygen to any part of your body can interfere with whatever happens to be going on there.

Before menopause, women should ordinarily be getting about 18 milligrams of iron a day. After menopause, 10 should be sufficient. This smaller amount is also applicable to men. It's likely that most of the iron in your diet is going to come from animal foods, but as you scan the table you'll notice that certain other foods, such as nuts, dried fruit and beans, have useful amounts of iron. Dairy products have virtually no iron at all. When eating a food that contains iron, particularly a vegetable food, it's an excellent idea to also eat a food that contains a goodly amount of vitamin C, because vitamin C can increase your absorption of iron from that food by 50 percent or more.

Vitamin A. A number of green leafy vegetables, fruits and root crops such as carrots and sweet potatoes contain very high amounts of vitamin A. But in looking at the table, you'll notice that there is a tendency for many foods to have a very low amount of this vitamin while a few have a very high amount. Therefore, it's possible that even someone eating a variety of foods could fail to get enough vitamin A.

A protective daily amount of this vitamin would be anything between 5,000 and 10,000 international units.

A deficiency of vitamin A will show itself in poor adaptability to dim light, poor resistance to infection, rough, bumpy skin and slow healing of wounds.

B vitamins. This category is a combination of thiamine (vitamin B_1) riboflavin (vitamin B_6), and niacin. Frequently, but not always, other B vitamins, such as B_6 and B_{12}, are found in foods that are rich in the other B vitamins as well. In those cases where foods are particularly good in one of the three major B vitamins but not in the others, I have tried to indicate that.

Vitamin C. Vitamin C has many functions, but perhaps its most basic one is in the creation of collagen, the body's connective tissue, which one researcher has compared to the reinforcing rods in cement. A deficiency of vitamin C or an exaggerated need for this nutrient can show itself in innumerable ways, including poor resistance to infection, bleeding gums and sores that fail to heal.

In general, it's safe to say that if you seek out foods that are rich in vitamin C, you'll be getting foods that are good for you for many other reasons as well, and that are generally quite low in calories.

There are many other important vitamins, minerals and food substances that I have not been able to include in this table. Vitamin E, vitamin D, magnesium, zinc and several B-vitamin factors are chief among the missing. Nevertheless, those presented here will at least give you some idea of what you're getting in the way of nutrition for the calories in many common foods.

Caloric equivalents and remarks. These entries will allow you to compare various foods for calorie content in a very rapid way. Usually I have listed similar foods or foods that might be eaten as substitutes. In many cases, I have also included dissimilar foods to give you some idea of the caloric relationship between "meal" foods and snack foods.

This section of the table will, I hope, be especially valuable in encouraging you to think more about your alternatives in meal planning, so that you can create meals that are very pleasing to your palate while having somewhat fewer calories than you ordinarily eat. The information will also be helpful in enabling you to analyze the caloric input of the various components of such popular combinations as a bacon-and-egg breakfast or a cheeseburger. With this knowledge, you can continue pretty much eating the kinds of dishes you want, if you reduce the calorie content by manipulating secondary components. You'll discover, for instance, that eating a cheeseburger without the bun will save 120 calories, while omitting the cheese instead will save almost as much—105 calories. But you can also find out that the cheese gives you twice as much protein and six times more calcium.

FOOD RATING AND EVALUATION TABLE

Food	Portion	Calories	N/C Rating	Protein (g.)	Calcium (mg.)
Almonds, shelled	½ oz. (about 11)	85	Good (if not abused)	2.6 (good)	33
Amaranth (cultivated *Amaranthus hypochondriacus*)					
Raw greens	2 oz. (1 cup chopped)	20 (estimated)	Excellent	1.9	151
Grains	1 oz.	109	Excellent	4.3 (excellent)	137
Apple	1 medium	80	Fair	0.3 (scant)	10 (scant)

Food Rating and Evaluation Guide

You'll discover that although cashew nuts are usually thought of as being very fattening, you're probably better off serving them at a party than potato chips, because each chip has the same number of calories as two cashews.

The remarks that I make in this section of the table allow me to offer some helpful tips—and do a little preaching as well.

Iron (mg.)	Vitamin A (I.U.)	B vitamins (mg.)	Vitamin C (mg.)	Caloric Equivalents and Remarks
0.6 (very good)	0	Little	0	1 tbs. peanut butter; 3 Brazil nuts; 3 walnuts; 8 peanuts in shell; 4 dates; ½ cup milk. Main value is protein and iron. Roasting in oil increases calories only slightly. Never eat from can.
2.2	3,458 (excellent)	Scant	44 (excellent)	Cultivated amaranth greens may soon be a popular "health food," especially among home gardeners. The minerals, however, are not totally available for absorption. Similar to spinach and kale.
1.0	0	Little	Trace	Roasted amaranth grains are usually added to baked goods, or popped like corn. Good protein complement to wheat. More protein and iron than sesame seeds with one-third fewer calories.
0.4 (good)	120 (not much)	Scant	6 (fair)	¾ cup orange juice; 1 small banana; 1 large piece bread. A big apple may have 125 calories. Not as nutritious as bananas, apricots or oranges. Similar to pears.

(continued)

FOOD RATING AND EVALUATION TABLE—*Continued*

Food	Portion	Calories	N/C Rating	Protein (g.)	Calcium (mg.)
Apple juice	1 glass (6 fl. oz.)	87	Poor	0.2	11
Applesauce (sweetened)	½ cup	116	Poor	0.25 (scant)	5
Apricots					
Raw	3 (12/lb.)	55	Excellent	1.1	18
Dried	¼ cup	85	Excellent	2	25
Apricot nectar	1 glass (6 fl. oz.)	107	Good (if not abused)	0.6	17
Asparagus	4 (medium)	12	Superb	1.3	13 (scant)

Food Rating and Evaluation Guide

Iron (mg.)	Vitamin A (I.U.)	B vitamins (mg.)	Vitamin C (mg.)	Caloric Equivalents and Remarks
1.1 (excellent)	0	Scant	2 (scant)	1 glass orange juice, 1 apple. Only value is iron. Orange juice has 45 times more vitamin C. Bereft of fiber in apple. Not recommended as beverage for adults.
0.65 (very good)	50 (scant)	Scant	1.5 (scant)	1 large apple (which has 6 times more vitamin C); ½ cantaloupe with 1 oz. cottage cheese; 15 almonds. More than half the calories are from the added sugar. Unsweetened applesauce has only 50 calories per ½ cup.
0.5	2,890 (excellent)	Scant (fair niacin)	11 (good)	1 very large peach; 1 wedge honeydew; 1 small orange. A very economical source of vitamins A and C and iron. One-half cup of apricots in heavy syrup has twice the calories, half the vitamin C.
2.1	4,090 (excellent)	Scant (fair niacin)	5	2 peaches; 4 prunes; ¼ cup raisins. Rich in iron, vitamin A, fiber. Never eat from box or bag; enjoy with fluid like herb tea.
0.4	1,790	Scant	6 (fair)	6 apricots; 1 large glass orange juice. High in vitamins but also high in fruit sugar. The whole fruit is far superior.
0.4	540 (good)	Little	16 (good)	About ¼ cup broccoli, spinach, or brussels sprouts. Almost calorie-free, they are worth their high price. Try adding raw to salads.

(continued)

FOOD RATING AND EVALUATION TABLE—*Continued*

Food	Portion	Calories	N/C Rating	Protein (g.)	Calcium (mg.)
Avocado	½	188	Fair to poor	2.4	11 (scant)
Bacon	2 medium slices	86	Fair	3.8 (good)	2
Banana	1 medium	101	Good	1.3	10
Beans, green (cooked quickly)	1 cup	31	Excellent	2	63
Beans, lima (cooked)	1 cup	189	Excellent	12.9 (excellent)	80
Beans, mung (sprouted, raw)	1 cup	37	Superb	4 (excellent)	20

Iron (mg.)	Vitamin A (I.U.)	B vitamins (mg.)	Vitamin C (mg.)	Caloric Equivalents and Remarks
0.7	330 (fair)	Fair	16 (good)	1 very large cantaloupe; 5 small peaches; 2 brownies. High in fat, avocados are best eaten only on special occasions, if at all. Melons are much better.
0.5 (good)	0	Scant	0	1 very small scrambled egg; 1 lightly buttered piece whole wheat toast; ⅔ cup oatmeal. Not as high in calories as you'd think, but preservative suspected of being dangerous.
0.8	230	Scant	12 (good)	2 medium peaches; 1 fairly large apple; 6 apricots; 1 brownie. A good source of iron, better than apples, but not as good as peaches or apricots on caloric basis.
0.8	680	Good	15	¾ cup broccoli or spinach. All green vegetables can and should be eaten freely as long as they are not lavishly buttered. Use vinegar and herbs, or eat raw in salad.
4.3	480	Good	29 (excellent)	1 small cup cooked lentils; ¾ cup brown rice; 1 cup mashed potatoes. Beans aren't "fattening"—a cup of limas has 40 fewer calories than a cup of cottage cheese, much more iron and fiber.
1.4	Scant	Good	20 (excellent)	Sprouts are 89% water, so you can see the rest of them is packed with vitamins, minerals, and protein. Load your salads, soups, and stews with these natural "vitamin pills." (See chapter 12.)

(continued)

FOOD RATING AND EVALUATION TABLE—*Continued*

Food	Portion	Calories	N/C Rating	Protein (g.)	Calcium (mg.)
Beans, navy					
Cooked (other white and red beans similar)	1 cup	224	Excellent	14.8 (excellent)	95 (good)
With pork and sweet sauce	1 cup	311	Very good	15.6 (excellent)	138 (very good)
Beef, corned	3 oz.	316	Fair to poor	19	8
Beef, ground					
Regular	3 oz.	245	Good	21	9
Lean	3 oz.	185	Very good	23	10
Beef, pot roast					
Lean and fat	6 oz.	490	Good (in moderation)	46	20

Iron (mg.)	Vitamin A (I.U.)	B vitamins (mg.)	Vitamin C (mg.)	Caloric Equivalents and Remarks
5.1 (excellent)	0	Good	0	1 hamburger (3 oz.); ⅔ cup chili con carne with beans; ½ cup macaroni and cheese; 1 cup brown rice. High in fiber, protein and minerals.
4.6 (excellent)	330	Fair to good	5	1 cup creamed chipped beef; 1½ cups cooked lentils; 2 cups cooked egg noodles; 1 peanut butter sandwich. Even with the high calories, delivers good nutrition and fills belly.
2.5	0	Excellent	0	Typical fatty delicatessen meat. Note that 3 times as much beef stew has one-third fewer calories. Corned beef (3 oz.) sandwich on rye with coleslaw has about 460 calories.
2.6	60	Excellent	0	4-plus oz. baked flounder; 2 jumbo scrambled eggs. A bun would add 120 calories; cheese, 100. Snacking on hamburgers is devastating.
3	20	Excellent	0	½ cup corned beef hash; 4 slices salami; 5 slices bologna; 1 hot dog. All lean beef is a good nutritional bargain but lacks fiber and vitamins A and C.
5.8 (excellent)	60 (scant)	Excellent (but all beef is weak in thiamine)	0	12 oz. broiled chicken; 10 oz. canned salmon; 9 oz. oil-pack tuna. This portion is average; many would eat 8 oz., some only 4.

(continued)

FOOD RATING AND EVALUATION TABLE—*Continued*

Food	Portion	Calories	N/C Rating	Protein (g.)	Calcium (mg.)
Beef, pot roast—*continued*					
Lean only	5 oz.	280	Very good	44	20
Beef, rib roast					
Lean and fat	6 oz.	750	Poor	34	16
Lean only	5.4 oz.	375	Very good	42	18
Beef, steak					
Broiled sirloin, lean and fat	6 oz.	660	Poor	40	18
Broiled sirloin, lean only	4 oz.	230	Excellent	36	14
Broiled round, lean and fat	6 oz.	440	Very good	48	20

Food Rating and Evaluation Guide

Iron (mg.)	Vitamin A (I.U.)	B vitamins (mg.)	Vitamin C (mg.)	Caloric Equivalents and Remarks
5.4	20	Excellent	0	Represents above piece of meat trimmed of all visible fat (not internal marbling). Note huge caloric savings. 2 oz. canned gravy would add about 50 calories.
4.4	140	Very good	0	4 3-oz. lean hamburgers; 13 oz. baked flounder; 11 slices whole wheat bread. This cut of meat is loaded with fat begging to be trimmed away (see below).
5.4	36	Excellent	0	1 cup creamed chipped beef; 1 cup pork and beans in tomato sauce; 1 piece chocolate cake. This cut represents about an 8-oz. serving of the above cut trimmed of fat. So although the original cut is larger, the calories are much reduced.
5	100	Excellent	0	10 oz. turkey potpie; 1½ grilled cheese sandwiches; 2 cups chili con carne with beans; 2 large pieces marble cake. Another fatty cut of meat.
4.4	20	Excellent	0	4 slices roast turkey; 1 cup cooked beans. This is the above cut trimmed of visible fat, which reduces the total fat by 85%, total calories 65%, size of serving 33%.
6	40	Excellent	0	1 cheeseburger; 8 oz. roast turkey; 12 oz. milk shake. Round steak is relatively lean, so even untrimmed of fat it's not bad.

(continued)

FOOD RATING AND EVALUATION TABLE—*Continued*

Food	Portion	Calories	N/C Rating	Protein (g.)	Calcium (mg.)
Beef, steak—*continued*					
Broiled round, lean only	4.8 oz.	260	Excellent	42	18
Beef and vegetable stew (home recipe, lean chuck)	1 cup (about 9 oz.)	218	Excellent	15.7	29
Beef potpie (home recipe)	1 piece (about 7.5 oz.)	517	Fair to poor	21.2	29
Beer. See Beverages, recreational					
Beets (cooked)	3 (2″ dia.)	45	Fair (poor if buttered)	1.5	21
Beverages, recreational					
Beer	1 bottle (12 oz.)	151	Very poor	1.1	18

Food Rating and Evaluation Guide

Iron (mg.)	Vitamin A (I.U.)	B vitamins (mg.)	Vitamin C (mg.)	Caloric Equivalents and Remarks
5	20	Excellent	0	A gram of protein here costs only 6 calories; a gram from fried chicken, 7; lean hamburger, 8; milk, 18; bacon, 22; liverwurst, 19; brownies, 95; raisins, 120.
2.9	2,400	Excellent	17	4 oz. lean sirloin; ½ cheeseburger; 4 oz. roast turkey; 10 thin pretzels. Combination of lean beef and vegetables is good; vegetables add vitamins and fiber to beef's protein. More filling than plain beef.
3.8	1,720	Excellent	6	Same quantity turkey potpie; nearly 10 oz. lean, broiled, round steak. Potpies are high in calories—but not as high as a Big Mac, with 540 calories.
0.75	30	Scant	9	1 cup cooked, diced carrots; ½ cup cooked parsnips; 1 heaping cup cooked, diced turnips. Carrots most nutritious.
Trace	0	Scant (some useful niacin)	0	1 12-oz. Coke; 1½ jiggers whiskey; 1 wineglass sweet wine; 14 large cashews; 3 chocolate chip cookies; 14 potato chips; 7 thin pretzels; 2 cups buttered popcorn.

(continued)

FOOD RATING AND EVALUATION TABLE—*Continued*

Food	Portion	Calories	N/C Rating	Protein (g.)	Calcium (mg.)
Beverages, recreational—*continued*					
Whiskey, gin, rum, vodka, etc.	1 jigger (1½ fl. oz.)	97 (80 proof) 105 (86 proof)	Worst	0	0
Wine, dessert (e.g., port)	1 wine-glass (3½ oz.)	141	Worst	0	0
Wine, table (e.g., Chablis)	1 wine-glass (3½ oz.)	87	Worst	0	0
Soda					
Club	1 bottle (12 oz.)	0	Worst	0	0
Cola	1 bottle (12 oz.)	144	Worst	0	0
Cream	1 bottle (12 oz.)	160	Worst	0	0
Fruit flavor	1 bottle (12 oz.)	171	Worst	0	0
Ginger ale	1 bottle (12 oz.)	113	Worst	0	0
Tonic (quinine)	1 bottle (12 oz.)	113	Worst	0	0

Iron (mg.)	Vitamin A (I.U.)	B vitamins (mg.)	Vitamin C (mg.)	Caloric Equivalents and Remarks
0	0	0	0	Many liquors once sold 86 proof are now changing to 80 proof. The caloric difference is minimal. Flavored liqueurs average 135 calories per jigger; creme de menthe or cacao, 150. Brandy and cognac same as whiskey.
0.4	0	0	0	1 bottle beer; 1 12-oz. Coke; 1¼ oz. cheddar cheese. One glass of port wine in lieu of dessert while dining out is okay; sipping sweet wine every day can be very fattening.
0.4	0	0	0	A bit more than half a bottle of beer or Coke; 1 glass apple juice. Not as sweet as dessert wine, not as filling as beer, not as hard as liquor, table wine is easily abused.
0	0	0	0	1 bottle of cream or cherry soda has more calories than a bottle of beer. But even 1 bottle of ginger ale a day consumed as an addition to maintenance-level calories would create 8 lb. of fat. Drinking anything except club soda with whiskey is especially dangerous for those with blood sugar problems. Very heavy soda consumption has been tentatively linked with occasional urinary irritation, even bleeding. Diet soda not recommended because of chemical sweeteners. Other caloric values (per 12-oz. serving): bitter lemon, 192; Gatorade, 60; Collins mixer, 128; Dr. Pepper, 132; ginger beer, 144; Wink, 178, Fruit "crush" drinks range up to 204 calories per 12 oz.
0	0	0	0	
0	0	0	0	
0	0	0	0	
0	0	0	0	
0	0	0	0	

(continued)

FOOD RATING AND EVALUATION TABLE–*Continued*

Food	Portion	Calories	N/C Rating	Protein (g.)	Calcium (mg.)
Biscuits (home recipe)	2 (2″ × 1¼″)	206	Fair to poor (if buttered)	4.2	68
Blueberries					
Raw	½ cup	45	Very good	0.5	11
Frozen, sweetened	½ cup	121	Fair to poor	0.7	7
Bluefish (broiled or baked with butter)	6 oz.	270	Excellent	44.4	48
Bologna	2 oz. (2 to 3 slices)	170	Fair to poor	6.7	3.9
Boston brown bread	1 piece (3¼″ × ½″)	95	Fair to poor (with cream cheese)	2.5	41

Food Rating and Evaluation Guide

Iron (mg.)	Vitamin A (I.U.)	B vitamins (mg.)	Vitamin C (mg.)	Caloric Equivalents and Remarks
0.8	0	Scant	0	A pat of butter on each of these 2 biscuits raises the caloric count to 278—more than 2 cupcakes and as much as a piece of marble cake. If you use buttered biscuits to sponge up gravy, you'd be better off getting the gravy with a spoon and eating cake for dessert.
0.75	75	Scant	10	½ banana or ½ large apple; 1 chocolate chip cookie; 1 fig bar. A good dessert or snack, with useful iron and vitamin C.
0.45	35	Scant	9	2 large wedges honeydew; 25 raw cherries or a little over ½ cup of cherries in syrup. Note decline in minerals and vitamins as calories go up—typical of what food processing does.
1.2	60	Very good	0	Curiously, has 20% fewer calories than baked flounder. Same calories as 5 oz. lean pot roast or 1 small hamburger. Fresh bluefish is one of the best-tasting of all fish; many meat lovers will enjoy its relatively robust flavor.
1	0	Fair	0	Ounce for ounce the same as regular hamburger, but hamburger has 3 times the protein, 2½ times the iron, more vitamins. Bologna is about one-quarter fat.
0.9	0	Little	0	1 brownie; 2 fig bars or chocolate chip cookies. Not too bad by itself (note high iron from molasses), if spread thickly with cream cheese, calories will easily double.

(continued)

FOOD RATING AND EVALUATION TABLE—*Continued*

Food	Portion	Calories	N/C Rating	Protein (g.)	Calcium (mg.)
Bouillon	1 cube	6 (see Remarks)	Good to poor	0.62	N/A*
Bran	N/A	N/A	N/A	N/A	N/A
Brazil nuts	6 large (1 oz.)	185	Fair (if not abused)	4.1	53
Bread					
Italian ("enriched")	1 medium slice (⅔ oz.)	56	Poor	1.8	4
Rye	1 slice (a bit less than 1 oz.)	61	Poor	2.3	19
White ("enriched")	1 slice (1 oz.)	76	Poor	2.4	24

*N/A = not available

Food Rating and Evaluation Guide

Iron (mg.)	Vitamin A (I.U.)	B vitamins (mg.)	Vitamin C (mg.)	Caloric Equivalents and Remarks
0.08	N/A	Little	N/A	How can you go wrong with a 5-calorie cup of hot broth? Easy—if it ignites your appetite instead of easing it. Loaded with salt.
N/A	N/A	N/A	N/A	Bran contains calories and other nutrients but adults are not ordinarily able to digest and utilize any significant amount. Young people can absorb at least some of these nutrients. Bran cereals often have added sugar.
1	0	High in niacin	0	18 peanuts in shell; 9 dates. Nuts are nutritious and high in zinc, but generous snacking is ill-advised.
0.4	0	Scant	0	Ounce for ounce, most breads are similar in calories. Moral: Eat smaller slices. Case in point: 1 hoagie roll has 392 calories.
0.4	0	Scant	0	Rye bread is made with just one-third rye flour and is similar to white bread in nutritive value. Pumpernickel has about twice as much iron and 4 times the potassium for same calories/oz.
0.7	0	Little	0	You may end up eating twice as much to satisfy your appetite. Not as chewy as whole wheat bread, it turns to paste when toasted and buttered, or in a sandwich with catsup. A sandwich of whole wheat bread will take longer to eat and leave you feeling more satisfied than one with white bread.

(*continued*)

FOOD RATING AND EVALUATION TABLE—*Continued*

Food	Portion	Calories	N/C Rating	Protein (g.)	Calcium (mg.)
Bread—*continued*					
Whole wheat	1 slice (1 oz.)	67	Good	2.6	24
Bread stuffing	½ cup	208	Poor	4.4	40
Broccoli (cooked stalks, cut into small pieces)	1 cup	40	Excellent	4.8	136
Brussels sprouts (boiled)	½ cup	28	Excellent	3.3	25
Butter	1 pat	36	Poor	0	1
Cabbage (cooked wedges)	1 cup	31	Excellent	1.7	71

Food Rating and Evaluation Guide

Iron (mg.)	Vitamin A (I.U.)	B vitamins (mg.)	Vitamin C (mg.)	Caloric Equivalents and Remarks
0.8	0	Good	0	Big bread eaters will save themselves a few pounds a year by eating whole wheat bread instead of white. More important, whole wheat has B vitamins and minerals not restored to "enriched" white and 8 times more fiber.
1	440	Little	0	1 full cup mashed potatoes made with butter; 2 biscuits (no butter). Adding gravy with fat drippings adds a lot more calories. Reserve for Thanksgiving and Christmas.
1.2	3,880	Excellent	140 (excellent)	1 dozen cooked, medium asparagus spears; 1⅓ cups green beans. Your best bet in green vegetables. It would be hard to find any food with more nutrition per calorie. Steam quickly.
0.85	405	Good to excellent	68 (excellent)	Another fine green vegetable. Avoid drenching with butter. Try lemon juice, herbs, or adding to stews.
0	170	0	0	Except for vitamin A, an empty-calorie food which is 80% pure fat. A 4-oz. stick of butter has 812 calories. Try to warm butter before serving so it can be spread thinly. One less pat a day means 4 lb. saved in a year.
0.5	200	Scant	41	A good way to add some bulk to a meal but not as nourishing as broccoli or brussels sprouts. Avoid drenching in butter. (See also Coleslaw.)

(continued)

FOOD RATING AND EVALUATION TABLE—*Continued*

Food	Portion	Calories	N/C Rating	Protein (g.)	Calcium (mg.)
Cakes					
Boston cream pie	1 small piece (see Remarks)	208	Poor	6.5	46
Chocolate (with icing)	1 small piece	277	Poor	3.4	53
Cupcake (chocolate icing)	1 (2½" dia.)	132	Poor	1.5	23
Fruitcake	1 slice (½" thick, about 1 oz.)	114	Poor	1.4	22
Gingerbread	1 piece (3" × 3" × 2")	371	Poor	4.4	80
Pound cake	1 slice (1 oz.)	142	Poor (probably worst cake)	1.7	6
Sponge cake	1 large piece (a little over 2 oz.)	196	Poor	5	20

Food Rating and Evaluation Guide

Iron (mg.)	Vitamin A (I.U.)	B vitamins (mg.)	Vitamin C (mg.)	Caloric Equivalents and Remarks
0.3	140	Scant	0	4 chocolate chip cookies; ½ cup bread stuffing. Important: a "small" piece is $\frac{1}{12}$ the cake. For a larger piece, ⅛ cake, add one-third more calories. A large piece of Boston cream pie, for example, has 311 calories.
0.8	120	Scant	0	2¾ brownies; 1 large cup ice cream. A large piece, the kind most men would eat, is 365 calories.
0.2	60	Scant	0	Equivalent to about ½ small piece chocolate cake.
0.8	40	Scant	0	1 large brownie; 1½ oz. raisins. This slice of fruitcake weighs less than half as much as the chocolate cake above. Ounce for ounce, there's not that much difference.
2.7 (excellent)	110	Little	0	1 large piece chocolate cake; 3 cupcakes. Topped with whipped cream, the calories hit 400.
0.2	80	Scant	0	This is a modest piece. Ounce for ounce, has more calories than chocolate cake. You might be happier making chocolate cake in loaf form and serving small slices.
0.8	300	Scant	0	Generally an especially poor choice because it doesn't satisfy a sweet tooth like other cakes.

(continued)

FOOD RATING AND EVALUATION TABLE–*Continued*

Food	Portion	Calories	N/C Rating	Protein (g.)	Calcium (mg.)
Candy, assorted	Candy has so little nutritional value there is no point in spelling out the minor differences. Here are calorie counts for 1 oz.: butterscotch, 113; caramels, 113; bittersweet chocolate, 135; milk chocolate, 147 (size of typical chocolate bar); vanilla cream, 123; chocolate fudge, 113; gum drops, 98; jelly beans, 104; marshmallows (4), 90. The grand champion is Reese's Peanut Butter Cups, one package of which, at just 1.2 ounces, has 190 calories. If you're "addicted" to candy, trying to eat smaller portions probably won't work. Better to exclude it completely.				
Cantaloupe	½ melon	82	Excellent	1.9	38
Carrots					
Raw	1 carrot	30	Excellent	0.8	27
Cooked and sliced	½ cup	24	Excellent	0.7	26
Casaba melon	1 wedge	38	Excellent	1.7	20
Cashew nuts (roasted in oil)	1 oz. (about 14 large kernels)	159	Fair (if not abused)	4.9	11
Catsup	1 tbs.	16	Good (as condiment)	0.3	3

Iron (mg.)	Vitamin A (I.U.)	B vitamins (mg.)	Vitamin C (mg.)	Caloric Equivalents and Remarks
1.1	9,240 (outstanding)	Good	90 (excellent)	Most people eat only half this much but when ½ cantaloupe has fewer calories than 1 piece of buttered toast, why stint?
0.5	7,930 (outstanding)	Scant	6	1 small wedge cantaloupe; 2 small apricots. A great source of vitamin A and a good source of fiber.
0.45	8,140 (outstanding)	Scant	5	Serve carrots as a side vegetable with both lunch and dinner. They're inexpensive, easy to prepare, and so low in calories you can eat giant helpings.
0.6	40	Little	18	Ounce for ounce, slightly fewer calories than cantaloupe. But they are poorer in vitamins and higher in price.
1.1	30	Good for niacin	0	18 roasted almonds; 5 Brazil nuts; 15 peanuts in shell; 1½ tbs. peanut butter. Party tip: 1 potato chip has same calories as 1 cashew.
0.1	210	Scant	2	The important thing about catsup is that it has 85 fewer calories than mayonnaise and 58 less than tartar sauce per tbs. Remember when eating sandwiches and fried fish.

(continued)

FOOD RATING AND EVALUATION TABLE—*Continued*

Food	Portion	Calories	N/C Rating	Protein (g.)	Calcium (mg.)
Cauliflower (cooked)	½ cup	14	Excellent	1.5	13
Celery	1 large stalk	7	Excellent	0.4	16
Cheese					
American	1 slice (1 oz.)	105	Good	6.6	198
Blue or Roquefort	1 oz.	104	Fair	6.1	89
Camembert	1 oz.	85	Poor (has little calcium)	5	30
Cheddar	1 oz. (2 small slices)	113	Good (if not abused)	7.1	213
Cottage (creamed)	6 oz.	180	Excellent	23	160
Swiss	Rectangular slice (1¼ oz.)	130	Very good	9.6	324 (outstanding)

Food Rating and Evaluation Guide

Iron (mg.)	Vitamin A (I.U.)	B vitamins (mg.)	Vitamin C (mg.)	Caloric Equivalents and Remarks
0.45	40	Little	35 (very good)	Another nutritious vegetable that can be eaten freely. Even when the price is high, cost of each serving is still only a few cents. Alternates are carrots, green beans, cabbage.
0.1	110	Scant	4	Although nearly calorie-free, observe whether snacking on celery calms or excites your appetite. Use generously in salads.
0.3	350	Very little	0	The blandness of American cheese makes it too easy to eat too much too fast. A bologna and cheese sandwich has 400 to 500 calories.
0.1	350	Good riboflavin	0	5 oz. milk; 1 slice American cheese. Cheese should be considered a meal food or dessert, not a snack—except for growing children.
0.1	290	Good riboflavin	0	The wedge that comes 3 to a 4-oz. box has 114 calories. When eating cheese, add 9 calories for each Wheat Thin, 22 for each Triscuit.
0.3	370	Good riboflavin	0	Best way to eat cheddar is to melt 1 slice over vegetables.
0.5	290	Excellent riboflavin	0	1½ 8-oz. containers of plain yogurt; 9 oz. milk; ⅔ container of yogurt with sweetened fruit. Cottage cheese has 3 times as much protein as yogurt ounce for ounce but about 20% less calcium.
0.3	400	Very little	0	The most nutritious popular cheese, though Parmesan has a bit more protein and excellent riboflavin.

(continued)

FOOD RATING AND EVALUATION TABLE—*Continued*

Food	Portion	Calories	N/C Rating	Protein (g.)	Calcium (mg.)
Cherries, sweet (raw)	10	47	Excellent	0.9	15
Chicken					
Roasted, white meat only	8 oz.	413	Excellent	72	25
Roasted, all flesh, skin and giblets	8 oz.	549	Excellent	61.7	27
Fried (including bone)	½ breast, 2 drumsticks (7.5 oz.)	335	Excellent	49	21
Chicken à la king (home recipe)	1 cup	468	Excellent	27.4	127
Chicken fricassee (home recipe)	1 cup	386	Excellent	36.7	14

Food Rating and Evaluation Guide

Iron (mg.)	Vitamin A (I.U.)	B vitamins (mg.)	Vitamin C (mg.)	Caloric Equivalents and Remarks
0.3	70	Scant	7	½ large apple; ½ banana; 3 small apricots. Even if you go berserk eating raw cherries you can't do too much damage. But ½ cup of cherries in syrup has 104 calories.
3	250	Excellent (superhigh in niacin)	0	4½ oz. lean and fat pot roast; 7 oz. lean hamburger. Chicken (minus fatty skin) is as economic a source of protein as lean-only round steak: about 6 calories per gram. Some people would eat less than the 8 oz. shown here.
4.6	1,790	Excellent (higher in thiamine and ribo-flavin than white)	0 (meat only)	Dark meat has only about 5% more calories than white; the difference here comes from skin and giblets. Nutrition balance better than white meat. Avoid skin but eat liver.
3.1	170	Excellent (but less than roasted)	0	Excluding bone, this is 5.3 oz. of meat, considerably less than above serving. 8 oz. of meat would have 500 calories.
2.5	1,130	Excellent	12	1 cup over 2 pieces of toast would go over 600 calories, but this is good nourishment. ½ cup over toast with fruit for dessert makes a good lunch.
2.2	170	Excellent	0	¾ cup chicken a la king; 6 oz. lean hamburger. Almost any way you fix chicken, the result is good nutrition.

(continued)

FOOD RATING AND EVALUATION TABLE—*Continued*

Food	Portion	Calories	N/C Rating	Protein (g.)	Calcium (mg.)
Chicken and noodles (home recipe)	1 cup	367	Very good	22.3	26
Chili con carne (with beans)	1 cup	339	Excellent	19.1	82
Chocolate. See Candy, assorted					
Cocoa (in a cup of water)	1 oz.	102	Fair	5.3	167
Coleslaw (made with commercial French dressing)	1 cup	114	Poor	1.4	50
Cookies					
Assorted	6	250	Poor	2.7	19

Iron (mg.)	Vitamin A (I.U.)	B vitamins (mg.)	Vitamin C (mg.)	Caloric Equivalents and Remarks
2.2	430	Very good	0	6 oz. lean ground beef; 7 oz. roasted white meat chicken. The noodles lower the protein density but you may find them nicely filling.
4.3	150	Very good	0	Equal to 1 Swiss cheese sandwich or ⅔ cup chicken a la king in both protein and calories. Other caloric equivalents: 1 piece apple pie; 2 doughnuts; ¾ cup macaroni and cheese; 5 oz. lean rib roast. With ½ cup brown rice, very filling, with fewer calories than beef potpie.
0.5	10	Good ribo-flavin only	1	If you use milk instead of water, the calorie count goes up to about 240, making a good drink for those who wish to gain weight. The caffeine, sugar, chocolate, and milk make this a doubtful beverage for sensitive children.
0.5	30	Scant	35	½ cup potato salad; 3½ cups green beans; 1 pound plain cooked cabbage. With mayonnaise instead of French dressing, calories go up about 60 points.
0.4	42	Scant	0	For about the same calories you could have (*a*) a carton of yogurt with fruit; (*b*) a wedge of cheddar cheese, 4 Wheat Thins, an apple, and a cup of coffee with milk; or (*c*) a bottle of beer and a dozen roasted almonds. So why eat cookies?

(continued)

FOOD RATING AND EVALUATION TABLE—*Continued*

Food	Portion	Calories	N/C Rating	Protein (g.)	Calcium (mg.)
Cookies—*continued*					
Brownies with nuts (home recipe)	1 (about 3″ × 3″ × 1″)	97	Poor	1.3	8
Chocolate chip (home recipe)	1	51	Poor	0.6	7
Fig bars	1	50	Poor	0.6	11
Gingersnaps	1	29	Poor	0.4	5
Macaroons	1	90	Poor	1	5
Marshmallow	1	74	Poor	0.7	4
Oatmeal with raisins	1	59	Poor	0.8	3
Oreo-type	1	50	Poor	0.5	3
Raisin	1 biscuit-type	67	Poor	0.8	13
Sugar wafers	1 large	44	Poor	0.4	0.3
Vanilla wafers	1 large	19	Poor	0.2	0.2

Iron (mg.)	Vitamin A (I.U.)	B vitamins (mg.)	Vitamin C (mg.)	Caloric Equivalents and Remarks
0.4	40	Scant	0	Brownies come in close to sugar and vanilla wafers in race for world's worst junk food.
0.4	20	Scant	0	
0.15	15	Scant	0	Fig bars sound more healthful than chocolate chip cookies, but you can see there's no real difference. The same goes for oatmeal-raisin cookies.
0.16	5	Scant	0	
0.15	0	Scant	0	
0.1	98	Scant	0	
0.37	7	Scant	0	
0.07	0	Scant	0	6 of these have as many calories as a 3-oz. lean hamburger on a bun with tomato, lettuce, and catsup. Which do you want?
0.37	38	Scant	0	If you must have cookies around the house for the kids, these would be a good choice.
0.03	13	Scant	0	Eating a sugar wafer is like eating 3 teaspoons of plain sugar.
0.02	5	Scant	0	In a dead heat with sugar wafers for the world's worst junk food.

(continued)

FOOD RATING AND EVALUATION TABLE—*Continued*

Food	Portion	Calories	N/C Rating	Protein (g.)	Calcium (mg.)
Corn					
Cooked on cob	1 ear	70	Very good	2.5	2
Canned	½ cup	70	Good	2.2	4
Crab, deviled	1 cup (about 8 oz.)	451	Good	27.4	113
Crackers					
Butter	5 large	87	Poor	1.4	28
Cheese (145/lb.)	10	150	Poor	3.5	105
Graham	1 large rectangular piece	55	Poor	1.1	6
Saltines (160/lb.)	4 singles	48	Poor	1	2

Food Rating and Evaluation Guide

Iron (mg.)	Vitamin A (I.U.)	B vitamins (mg.)	Vitamin C (mg.)	Caloric Equivalents and Remarks
0.5	310	Good niacin	7	½ baked potato; 2 cups green beans; ½ small piece corn bread. Brush lightly with melted butter, or rub quickly with butter stick to reduce calories.
0.4	290	Some niacin	4	See above for equivalents. Loses B vitamins and half of vitamin C in canning process—along with taste.
2.9	0	Very good	14	10 oz. canned salmon; 9 oz. broiled swordfish. (Some would eat about one-third less than amount of deviled crab in chart.) Plain crab has only about half the calories per oz. and more protein, but who can afford it?
0.1	40	Scant	0	1 small brownie; 11 almonds; 1 apple; 1 glass apple juice. Not much here except calories. Eating these 5 crackers every day in addition to your maintenance calories will add 10 pounds in a year.
0.3	110	Scant	0	10 crackers weigh 1⅓ oz.—that much cheddar has same calories but 3 times as much protein and calcium and 5 times more vitamin A.
0.2	0	Scant	0	"Graham" cracker has healthful connotations but it is basically a sugar biscuit.
0.1	0	0	0	For another 20 calories you could have a piece of whole wheat bread with your soup and get some honest nourishment while you're at it.

(continued)

FOOD RATING AND EVALUATION TABLE—*Continued*

Food	Portion	Calories	N/C Rating	Protein (g.)	Calcium (mg.)
Crackers—*continued*					
Cheese-peanut butter sandwiches	4 (1 packet, 1 oz.)	139	Poor	4.3	16
Cranberry Juice Cocktail	1 glass (6 fl. oz.)	124	Fair to poor	0.2	10
Cream, light (see also Sour cream; Toppings, whipped)	1 tbs.	32	Poor	0.5	15
Cream, whipped	½ cup	209	Poor	1.3	45
(from heavy whipping cream)	1 tbs.	27	Poor	0.15 (scant)	6
Cream puff	1	303	Poor	8.5	105
Cucumber (with skin)	1 small	25	Excellent	1.5	42
Custard, baked	1 cup	305	Fair (if not abused)	14.3	297

Food Rating and Evaluation Guide

Iron (mg.)	Vitamin A (I.U.)	B vitamins (mg.)	Vitamin C (mg.)	Caloric Equivalents and Remarks
0.2	10	A little niacin	0	Popular vending machine item packs a surprising caloric punch, virtually same as a chocolate bar.
0.6	0	Scant	30	1½ glasses orange juice; 3 oz. cranberry sauce; 2 large peaches; 2 oranges. The orange juice has 3 times more vitamin C. Two-thirds of the calories here are from added sugar.
0	130	Trace	0	Using this instead of milk for your coffee adds about 20 calories per cup. Other values per tbs.—half-and-half, 20; light whipping, 45; heavy whipping, 53.
Scant	917	Some riboflavin	Scant	2 brownies; small piece Boston cream pie; 1 10-oz. glass milk. Can easily be abused.
Scant	115	Trace	0	1 small pat of butter or margarine; 1 gingersnap; 1 marshmallow.
0.9	460	Good riboflavin	0	1 heaping cup ice cream; 3 brownies; 1 medium piece chocolate cake; 2 bottles beer—any of which would probably be more satisfying.
1.9	420	Little	19	1 carrot; 1 green pepper. You'll lose 75% of that terrific iron value if you pare the cucumber. Grow your own to avoid the wax.
1.1	930	Excellent riboflavin	1	2 glasses milk; 3 scrambled eggs; 1 cream puff. A good food for slender children and convalescents. an occasional ½ cup for adults pays for itself with protein and calcium.

(continued)

FOOD RATING AND EVALUATION TABLE—*Continued*

Food	Portion	Calories	N/C Rating	Protein (g.)	Calcium (mg.)
Dates (with pits)	5	110	Poor	0.9	24
Doughnut	1 medium (3¼″ dia.)	164	Poor	1.9	17
Eggplant (cooked and diced)	1 cup	38	Excellent	2	22
Eggs					
Hard-boiled	1 large	82	Excellent	6.5 (excellent)	27
Scrambled	1 large	111	Excellent	7.2 (excellent)	51
"Fast foods"					

Iron (mg.)	Vitamin A (I.U.)	B vitamins (mg.)	Vitamin C (mg.)	Caloric Equivalents and Remarks
1.2	20	Some niacin	0	¼ cup dried apricots; 1 oz. raisins; 14 almonds. Unless you can be satisfied eating 2 or 3 as a snack, better avoid.
0.6	30	Little	0	1 bagel; 1 piece corn bread; 1 pancake; 1 hard roll; 1 plain Danish. Just 1 a week over maintenance will add a pound in 6 months.
1.2	20	Good for calorie cost	6	¼ baked potato; 1 large cup cabbage; ¾ cup brussels sprouts. An excellent vegetable which tends to block absorption of cholesterol eaten at same time, as from cheese.
1.2 (excellent)	590	Good riboflavin	0	An egg is one of the few foods that can be boiled without losing nutrients. Protein here costs only 12.6 calories per gram (you need about 60 to 70 grams a day). By comparison, lean round steak or broiled halibut costs 6; cheddar cheese, 16; milk, 18; white bread, 32.
1.1 (excellent)	690	Good riboflavin	0	This assumes addition of some butter and milk to above egg, adding about 30 calories. Even so, nutritional value is still excellent for calorie cost.
				Fast foods are often high in protein, calcium and B vitamins, but low in vitamin A, fiber and minerals. If you eat a lot of fast foods, you should try to supplement your diet with fresh vegetables, fruits, whole grain breads and cereals, and dairy products.

(continued)

FOOD RATING AND EVALUATION TABLE—*Continued*

Food	Portion	Calories	N/C Rating	Protein (g.)	Calcium (mg.)
"Fast foods"—*continued*					
McDonald's	All "fast foods"—1 serving				
Hamburger		257	Good	13	63
Cheese-burger		306	Good	16	158
Quarter-pounder, plain		418	Good	26	79
Quarter-pounder, with cheese		518	Good	31	251
Big Mac		540	Fair	26	175
Filet-O-Fish		402	Fair	15	105
French fries		211	Poor	3.1	10
Chocolate shake		364	Poor	10.7	338
Vanilla shake		323	Poor	10	346
Apple pie		300	Poor	2.2	12
Cherry pie		298	Poor	2.2	11.6

Food Rating and Evaluation Guide

Iron (mg.)	Vitamin A (I.U.)	B vitamins (mg.)	Vitamin C (mg.)	Caloric Equivalents and Remarks
329	231	Excellent	1.8	
2.9	372	Excellent	1.6	
5	164	Excellent	2.3	
4.6	683	Excellent	2.9	
4.3	327	Excellent	2.4	Same amount of meat as Quarter-pounder but lots more calories.
1.8	152	Excellent	4.2	Fish is no caloric bargain at McDonald's, thanks to sauce. Has 33% more calories than cheeseburger; less iron and protein.
0.5	Scant	Good niacin	11	
1.0	318	Good	Scant	
0.2	346	Good	Scant	
0.6	Scant	Little	2.7	
0.4	213	Some niacin	1.3	

(continued)

FOOD RATING AND EVALUATION TABLE—*Continued*

Food	Portion	Calories	N/C Rating	Protein (g.)	Calcium (mg.)
"Fast foods"—*continued*					
McDonald's—*continued*					
Hot fudge sundae		290	Poor	6.2	180
Egg McMuffin		352	Fair	18	187
Hot cakes with butter and syrup		472	Poor	8	154
Hash-brown potatoes		130	Poor	1.3	8
Kentucky Fried Chicken	All "fast foods"—1 serving				
Fried chicken, mashed potatoes, coleslaw, roll					
3-piece dinner, original		830	Fair	52	N/A*
3-piece dinner, crispy		950	Fair	52	N/A
2-piece dinner, original		661	Fair	33	13

*N/A = not available

Food Rating and Evaluation Guide

Iron (mg.)	Vitamin A (I.U.)	B vitamins (mg.)	Vitamin C (mg.)	Caloric Equivalents and Remarks
0.5	290	Some niacin and riboflavin	Scant	
3.2	361	Good	1.6	
2.4	255	Good	Scant	
Scant	Scant	Good niacin	Scant	
N/A	N/A	N/A	N/A	Rating would be "good" except for coleslaw and rolls. "Crispy" adds 80 to 120 greasy calories but no protein.
N/A	N/A	N/A	N/A	
21	N/A	N/A	N/A	

(*continued*)

FOOD RATING AND EVALUATION TABLE—*Continued*

Food	Portion	Calories	N/C Rating	Protein (g.)	Calcium (mg.)
Kentucky Fried Chicken—*continued*					
Fried chicken—*continued*					
2-piece dinner, crispy		902	Fair	36	14
Burger King	All "fast foods"—1 serving				
Hamburger		310	Good	16	6
Double hamburger		520	Good	26	N/A
Whopper		670	Poor	27	10
Whopper Jr.		370	Good	16	6
French fries		210	Poor	3	N/A

*N/A = not available

Iron (mg.)	Vitamin A (I.U.)	B vitamins (mg.)	Vitamin C (mg.)	Caloric Equivalents and Remarks
36	N/A	Good thiamine, riboflavin, niacin, B_6 and B_{12}	N/A	
15	N/A	Good thiamine, riboflavin, niacin, B_6 and B_{12}	N/A	
N/A	N/A	N/A	N/A	
25	N/A*	Good thiamine, riboflavin, niacin, B_6 and B_{12}	N/A	The Whopper has 300 extra calories but only 5 grams of protein more than a double hamburger at the same restaurant.
15	N/A	Good thiamine, riboflavin, niacin, B_6 and B_{12}	N/A	
2	N/A	Good thiamine, riboflavin, niacin, B_6 and B_{12}	N/A	

(continued)

FOOD RATING AND EVALUATION TABLE—*Continued*

Food	Portion	Calories	N/C Rating	Protein (g.)	Calcium (mg.)
"Fast foods"—*continued*					
Burger King—*continued*					
Chocolate shake		383	Poor	10	32
Pizza Hut. See Pizza					
Figs	1 medium	40	Fair (if not abused)	0.6	18
Fish sticks (breaded)	6 (6 oz.)	300	Fair	28.2	18
Flounder (baked with butter)	6 oz.	342	Excellent	51	42
Gelatin dessert (made with water)	1 cup	142	Worst	3.6	0
Grapefruit	½	40	Excellent	0.5	16

Food Rating and Evaluation Guide

Iron (mg.)	Vitamin A (I.U.)	B vitamins (mg.)	Vitamin C (mg.)	Caloric Equivalents and Remarks
5	N/A	Good thiamine, riboflavin, niacin, B_6 and B_{12}	N/A	
0.3	40	Little	1	2 dates; 1 mouthful raisins. Slightly more nutritious than dates (per calorie) except for iron. Avoid eating from bag or carton.
0.6	0	Good niacin	0	6 oz. flounder; 3 fried fish cakes. Eating with 3 tbs. tartar sauce will add another 225 calories.
2.4	0	Excellent	6	7 fish sticks; 3 large fish cakes; 7½ oz. baked bluefish; 3 oz. lean and fat broiled sirloin. Note superiority in protein and iron to fish sticks. Better yet: You can enjoy flounder with lemon instead of tartar sauce usually used on fish sticks.
0	0	0	0	Same as typical candy bar except candy bars are slightly more nutritious. The protein here is poorly balanced and largely useless.
0.4	10 (white) 420 (pink)	Scant	37	½ glass orange juice; ¼ cantaloupe. A good breakfast fruit. For a snack, cut whole fruit in half and slice into wedges. A glass of grapefruit juice has a dozen less calories than orange juice; vitamin C identical.

(continued)

FOOD RATING AND EVALUATION TABLE—*Continued*

Food	Portion	Calories	N/C Rating	Protein (g.)	Calcium (mg.)
Grape juice (bottled)	1 glass (6 fl oz.)	125	Poor	0.4	21
Grapes, seedless	10	34	Fair	0.3	6
Halibut (broiled with butter)	6 oz.	288	Excellent	42.6	30
Honey	1 tbs.	64	Poor	0.1	1
Honeydew melon	1 small wedge (1/10 of melon)	49	Very good	1.2	21
Ice cream	1 slice or 1/2 cup (4 oz.)	127	Poor	3	96
Jams and preserves	1 tbs.	54	Poor	0.1	4

Food Rating and Evaluation Guide

Iron (mg.)	Vitamin A (I.U.)	B vitamins (mg.)	Vitamin C (mg.)	Caloric Equivalents and Remarks
0.6	0	Scant	0	A glance at the chart reveals that grape juice is basically sugar water with a good dose of iron. A glassful made from frozen concentrate has 99 calories. An easily abused beverage.
0.2	50	Scant	2	½ small apple; about a tsp. of raisins. (Raisins have a high sugar content and are too easy to eat.) A cup has 107 calories. Best nutrients iron and potassium.
1.2	1,140	High in niacin only	0	5 oz. broiled flounder; 4-plus oz. fried oysters.
0.1	0	Trace	0	Some may find that because of the stronger taste they can use less honey to sweeten than sugar. But a tbs. of sugar has only 46 calories.
0.6	60	Some niacin	34	1 very large wedge cantaloupe; 1 large wedge casaba melon; ½ very large grapefruit. Cantaloupe has less calories, twice the vitamin C, 100 times more vitamin A/calorie.
0	290	Some riboflavin	1	1 very small slice pizza; 1 cup buttered popcorn. Ice cream isn't the world's worst dessert—it has useful calcium and less calories than 6 thin pretzels, ⅓ cup chocolate pudding, 1 doughnut, or 1 Twinkie. All the same, keeping ice cream in the freezer can be hazardous to your hips.
0.2	0	0	0	A tbs. of sugar has 8 less calories. Buy kinds you don't really like and use very sparingly if at all.

(continued)

FOOD RATING AND EVALUATION TABLE—*Continued*

Food	Portion	Calories	N/C Rating	Protein (g.)	Calcium (mg.)
Kale (boiled)	½ cup	22	Excellent	2.5	103
Lamb chop (lean)	2 (thick, 5.2 oz. total meat)	280	Very good (when trimmed of fat)	42	18
Lemonade (made from frozen concentrate)	1 glass (6 fl. oz.)	81	Poor	0.1	2
Lentils (cooked)	1 cup	212	Excellent	15.6	50
Lettuce, iceberg	1 wedge (⅙ of head)	12	Excellent	0.8	18
Liver, beef (fried)	2 slices or 6 oz.	390	Excellent	44.8 (excellent)	18

Food Rating and Evaluation Guide

Iron (mg.)	Vitamin A (I.U.)	B vitamins (mg.)	Vitamin C (mg.)	Caloric Equivalents and Remarks
0.9	4,565	Useful	102	Another super-nutritious, nearly calorie-free green. Some prefer it to spinach because its calcium is more available. Extraordinary vitamins A and C.
3	0	Very good	0	Lamb can be a high-calorie food if you don't trim the fat. These chops, untrimmed, would total 800 calories, while 6 oz. of shoulder would be 570. Lean lamb is similar to very lean beef.
0.1	10	Scant	.13	1 glass orange juice; ½ cantaloupe, both of which are far superior nutritionally.
4.2	40	Good	0	1 cup cooked beans; 10 french fries. Lentils, like all legumes (e.g., peas, limas, beans) have solid protein, iron, B vitamins, fiber. They're also filling. Eat with grain product for best protein value.
0.5	300	Scant	5	The important thing about lettuce is what you dress it with. An entire head has the same calories as 1 tbs. Russian dressing.
15 (outstanding)	90,780 (outstanding)	Outstanding	46 (excellent)	6½ oz. lean ground beef; 4 oz. corned beef; 8 oz. roasted white meat chicken; 8 oz. broiled halibut; 4.5 oz. liverwurst. Liver is probably the most nutritious food you could eat. Especially good for chronic dieters short on B vitamins and iron.

(continued)

FOOD RATING AND EVALUATION TABLE—*Continued*

Food	Portion	Calories	N/C Rating	Protein (g.)	Calcium (mg.)
Liverwurst (fresh)	3 oz.	265	Good	14	8
Lobster (cooked)	1 cup of pieces (about 5 oz.)	138	Excellent	27.1	9.7
Macaroni and cheese	1 cup	430	Good	16.8	362
Mangos	1	152	Good	1.6	23
Margarine	1 pat	36	Poor	0	1
Marmalade	1 tbs.	51	Poor	0.1	7

Food Rating and Evaluation Guide

Iron (mg.)	Vitamin A (I.U.)	B vitamins (mg.)	Vitamin C (mg.)	Caloric Equivalents and Remarks
4.59	5,400	Outstand-ing	0	1 large hamburger; 2 large, lean lamb chops. Smoked liverwurst (braunschweiger) is similar. A good luncheon meat (most are poor), but avoid heavy use of mayonnaise.
1.2	0	Good thiamine	0	Because lobster is almost fat-free it has an exceptional calorie/protein ratio: only 5/g. But eating with 3 tbs. drawn butter raises calories to 444 and changes ratio to 16:1. 1 cup lobster Newberg has 485 calories; 1 cup lobster salad, 572.
1.8	860	Very good	0	4 scrambled eggs; 6 oz. broiled round; 2 cups of beef and vegeta-ble stew. 1 cup of the latter stew over ½ cup rice would save almost 100 calories, give far better nutri-tion (except calcium), and be just as filling.
0.9	11,090	Good	81	2 apples; 3 medium peaches. This is a high-calorie fruit with high levels of vitamins. Suitable for dessert but not as a regular snack.
0	170	0	0	Chemically manipulated to have same nutritional profile as butter. No advantage to the weight-conscious.
0.1	0	0	1	1 tbs. jam; 1½ pats butter. Here is an item worthy of total elimination from the diet. That 1-lb. jar in your refrigerator is 1,166 calories looking for a warm home.

(continued)

FOOD RATING AND EVALUATION TABLE—*Continued*

Food	Portion	Calories	N/C Rating	Protein (g.)	Calcium (mg.)
Mayonnaise	1 tbs.	101	Poor	0.2	3
Milk	1 glass (6 fl. oz.)	119	Good	6.4	216
Molasses, blackstrap	1 tbs.	43	Very good (as sweetener, in moderation)	0	137
Muffins, blueberry	1	112	Fair	2.9	34
Mushrooms	½ cup sliced	10	Excellent	1	2
Nectarines	1	88	Good	0.8	6
Noodles	½ cup	100	Fair	3.3	8

Food Rating and Evaluation Guide

Iron (mg.)	Vitamin A (I.U.)	B vitamins (mg.)	Vitamin C (mg.)	Caloric Equivalents and Remarks
0.1	40	0	0	No more nourishing than marmalade and has twice the calories. 1 cup has fat-power to add ½ lb. to your weight. Wean away from mayonnaise habit by cutting with increasing amount of catsup. Wherever possible, use yogurt instead.
0	263	Good riboflavin	2	4 oz. cottage cheese (which would have 3 times more protein). Over-rated as a protein source, milk has outstanding calcium, but Swiss cheese has one-third more per calorie. A glass of skim milk has 66 calories; low-fat, 109; buttermilk, 66.
3.2	0	Little	0	Add to half the above glass of milk and you get more total calcium for fewer calories than from a whole glass of milk, plus a sweet taste and a good shot of iron. Contains factors which help metabolize sugar.
0.6	90	Little	0	1 piece bread with 1 pat butter; 1 biscuit. If smeared with butter, rating would drop to poor.
0.3	0	Very good	1	Probably best way for weight-conscious to get iron and B vitamins. Although absolute amounts not in same league as meat, on calorie basis are outstanding for nutrients. Add to soups, stews, salads.
0.7	2,280	0	18	1 very large orange; 1 apple; ¼ avocado. More vitamin A and iron than an orange but less vitamin C. Too easy to eat too many.
0.7	55	Good	0	½ cup rice; ⅔ baked potato. Best eaten without butter, as a bed for stews, meat sauces.

(continued)

FOOD RATING AND EVALUATION TABLE—*Continued*

Food	Portion	Calories	N/C Rating	Protein (g.)	Calcium (mg.)
Oatmeal (cooked)	1 cup	132	Good	4.8	22
Oils (corn, safflower, etc.)	1 tbs.	120	Poor	0	0
Olives, mission	5 extra large	44	Poor	0.3	25
Onions (sliced, raw)	¼ cup	11	Excellent	0.4	8
Orange					
Whole	1 average size	65	Very good	1	54

Food Rating and Evaluation Guide

Iron (mg.)	Vitamin A (I.U.)	B vitamins (mg.)	Vitamin C (mg.)	Caloric Equivalents and Remarks
1.4	0	Little	0	Has only 20 calories more than 1 scrambled egg. Added milk compensates for lack of calcium, boosts vitamins A and B. Best thing about oatmeal is that it's filling. Try adding 1 tbs. bran.
0	0	0	0	About ¾ of a candy bar; 8 teaspoons of sugar. A small amount of vegetable oil is needed for health, but most get far more oil than required.
0.4	15	0	0	2 thin pretzels; 6 roasted almonds. A few olives as a garnish won't hurt unless you're seriously avoiding salt. But as a snack, the almonds are much better.
0.15	12	Scant	3	Why are onions an excellent condiment while olives are "poor"? For one thing, olives have 27 times more sodium (salt) than potassium; onions, 15 times more potassium than sodium. And onions—raw or cooked—help reduce high cholesterol.
0.5	260	Good niacin	66	¾ nectarine or apple; 1 very large wedge cantaloupe; ¾ of a whole grapefruit; ¾ glass of orange juice. The cantaloupe has similar vitamin C, more iron, much more vitamin A. A large navel orange has 87 calories, 105 mg. of vitamin C.

(continued)

FOOD RATING AND EVALUATION TABLE–*Continued*

Food	Portion	Calories	N/C Rating	Protein (g.)	Calcium (mg.)
Orange–*continued*					
Juice	1 glass (6 fl. oz.)	84	Very good	1.3	20
Oysters, raw	6 medium (3 oz.)	57	Excellent	7.2	81
Pancake (made from mix with milk and eggs)	1 (6″ dia.)	164	Fair to poor	5.3	157
Peaches					
Fresh	1 (about 2½ per lb.)	58	Excellent	0.9	14
Dried	5 large halves	190	Fair to poor	2.3	35

Food Rating and Evaluation Guide

Iron (mg.)	Vitamin A (I.U.)	B vitamins (mg.)	Vitamin C (mg.)	Caloric Equivalents and Remarks
.37	375	Good thiamine	93	A few more calories than grapefruit juice, a few less than apple juice. This portion is relatively large—in a restaurant you'd probably get 4 oz. Besides high vitamin C, oranges have good thiamine and folate, required for healthy nerves.
4.8	270	Good	0	With 3 tbs. cocktail sauce, calorie count goes to 115, about the same as a hard dinner roll and butter. These same oysters fried have 162 calories. A cup of oyster stew has about 220 calories and excellent nutritive values.
0.5	180	Good	0	The important thing about pancakes is what you eat them with. 2 pancakes with 3 tbs. syrup and 2 pats butter are good for 580 calories. Stick to eggs and lightly buttered toast—far more protein for about 200 calories less.
0.8	2,030	Good niacin	11	¾ apple or nectarine; 1 large wedge cantaloupe. Twice the iron and vitamin C of an apple, 17 times the vitamin A—for about 20 fewer calories. But eat the same peach canned in syrup and the calorie count shoots up to about 160. Peach nectar has 90 calories per glass and only 800 units of vitamin A.
4.4	2,830	Excellent niacin	13	A highly nutritious snack for slender people. But the nutrients come at too high a caloric price for you and me.

(continued)

Appendix D

FOOD RATING AND EVALUATION TABLE—*Continued*

Food	Portion	Calories	N/C Rating	Protein (g.)	Calcium (mg.)
Peanut butter	1 tbs.	94	Fair (in moderation)	4	9
Peanuts (roasted in shell)	10	105	Fair (in moderation)	4.7	13
Pear	1 Bartlett	100	Fair	1.1	13
Peas (cooked)	⅓ cup	41	Excellent	3	13
Pecans (250 or less/lb.)	10 halves	124	Poor	1.7	13
Pepper, green	1 large	36	Excellent	2	15

Food Rating and Evaluation Guide

Iron (mg.)	Vitamin A (I.U.)	B vitamins (mg.)	Vitamin C (mg.)	Caloric Equivalents and Remarks
0.3	0	Excellent niacin	0	3 walnuts; 2 slices salami. A peanut butter and jelly sandwich made with 3 tbs. peanut butter and 1 tbs. of jelly has 483 calories—as much as a large serving of meat. If you love peanut butter and can't help snacking on it, don't buy it.
0.4	0	Excellent niacin	0	14 almonds; 3 large walnuts; 1 large tbs. peanut butter. A nutritious snack in moderation. Always eat from shell. ½ cup salted peanuts has 421 calories. The 1-lb. bag of roasted nuts you bring home contains 1,769 calories.
0.5	30	Scant	7	1 large apple or nectarine. Similar to apple in nutritive value. A Bosc pear has an average 86 calories; a D'Anjou, 122. A pear canned in syrup has about 140 calories; 2 dried pear halves, 94.
0.9 (excellent)	287	Excellent	10	Another excellent vegetable. Like other legumes (beans, etc.) they're high in protein and iron, but also have very good vitamin values. Good for adding bulk to stews, so you don't have to butter them.
0.4	20	Good thiamine	0	12 peanuts in shell; 4 walnuts. Probably the least nutritious of all nuts—a very poor snack item.
1.1	690	Very good	210	Calorie for calorie, one of the most nutritious of all foods. As much iron as ½ cantaloupe, with twice the vitamin C. A stuffed pepper has 315 calories, 24 g. protein, 74 mg. vitamin C. Tip: Gardeners should let some green peppers ripen to red. Vitamin A value will explode to 7,300 and vitamin C to 335. Calories increase to 51.

(continued)

FOOD RATING AND EVALUATION TABLE—*Continued*

Food	Portion	Calories	N/C Rating	Protein (g.)	Calcium (mg.)
Pies					
Apple	1 small piece (⅛ pie)	302	Poor	2.6	9
Banana custard	1 small piece (⅛ pie)	252	Poor	5.1	75
Blueberry	1 small piece (⅛ pie)	286	Poor	2.8	13
Cherry	1 small piece (⅛ pie)	308	The pits	3.1	17
Coconut custard	1 small piece (⅛ pie)	268	Poor	6.8	107
Lemon meringue	1 small piece (⅛ pie)	268	Poor	3.9	15
Mince	1 small piece (⅛ pie)	320	Poor	3	33
Pecan	1 small piece (⅛ pie)	431	Poor	5.3	48

Food Rating and Evaluation Guide

Iron (mg.)	Vitamin A (I.U.)	B vitamins (mg.)	Vitamin C (mg.)	Caloric Equivalents and Remarks
0.4	40	Scant	1	3 large apples; 1 heaping cup ice cream. NOTE: Pies are so caloric that dimensions are critical. A "small" piece has a 3½″ arc. For large piece (4¾″ arc, ⅙ of pie) add one-third to calories. E.g., a large piece of apple pie has 404 calories.
0.6	290	Little	1	2½ bananas; 1 cup ice cream. A large piece has 336 calories.
0.7	40	Scant	4	3 cups raw blueberries. With 4 oz. of ice cream on top, good for 413 calories.
0.4	520	Scant	0	65 raw cherries; 6 chocolate chip cookies; 1 medium slice chocolate cake. The 45 mg. of vitamin C that would be in those 65 cherries have turned into nothing here—except sugar.
0.8	260	Good ribo-flavin only	0	If pie must be served, here's the one with the most protein and calcium, and some useful iron.
0.5	180	Scant	3	1 cup ice cream—which has 13 times more calcium; 25 roasted peanuts in shell.
1.2	0	Scant	1	A mince pie looks nourishing but isn't, except for the iron. It has poorer calorie/protein ratio than brownies.
2.9	160	Some thia-mine and niacin	0	Pecan pie takes the cake in the calorie department. A whole pie has 3,449 calories. 1 small piece with 4 oz. ice cream is good for 558 calories.

(continued)

FOOD RATING AND EVALUATION TABLE—*Continued*

Food	Portion	Calories	N/C Rating	Protein (g.)	Calcium (mg.)
Pies—*continued*					
Pumpkin	1 small piece (⅛ pie)	241	Poor (except on Thanksgiving)	4.6	58
Pineapple					
Raw	2 slices	88	Good	0.6	28
Canned, with syrup	2 slices	156	Poor	0.6	24
Pizza					
Homemade, with cheese topping	1 piece (⅛ of 14″ pizza; 5⅓″ arc)	153	Fair (in moderation)	7.8	144

Food Rating and Evaluation Guide

Iron (mg.)	Vitamin A (I.U.)	B vitamins (mg.)	Vitamin C (mg.)	Caloric Equivalents and Remarks
0.6	2,810	Some riboflavin	0	The high vitamin A looks like a good excuse until you remember that ½ cantaloupe has 3 times as much for only 82 calories. But enjoy pumpkin pie with an easy conscience on holidays.
0.8 (excellent)	120	Scant	28 (excellent)	1 nectarine; ½ cantaloupe. These slices are 3½″ diam. and ¾″ thick. Some pineapples are considerably wider. Unsweetened juice has 103 calories per glass.
0.6	100	Scant	14	A good example of what happens to fruit when canned in syrup; calories double while vitamins shrink. If canned in water without sugar, calories actually decrease slightly, probably as natural sugars in raw fruit are lost. Vitamin C is also lost.
0.7	410	Good riboflavin	5	The problem with pizza is that a whole one (14″ diam.) has 1,227 calories and half of that is 614. That's not excessive if you have pizza for dinner, because it does have excellent protein, iron and calcium. But as a late-night snack, half a pizza is brutal.

(continued)

FOOD RATING AND EVALUATION TABLE—*Continued*

Food	Portion	Calories	N/C Rating	Protein (g.)	Calcium (mg.)
Pizza—*continued*					
Pizza Hut	½ 13″ pizza (3 slices)				
Thin crust					
Plain		680	Fair	38	100
Beef		490	Fair	29	N/A
Pork		520	Fair	27	N/A
Cheese		450	Fair	25	N/A
Pepperoni		430	Fair	23	N/A
Supreme		800	Fair	42	80
Thick crust					
Beef		620	Fair	38	N/A*
Pork		640	Fair	36	N/A
Cheese		560	Fair	34	N/A
Pepperoni		560	Fair	31	N/A
Supreme		640	Fair	36	N/A
Plums	1 (2⅛″ dia.)	32	Excellent	0.3	8

*N/A = not available

Iron (mg.)	Vitamin A (I.U.)	B vitamins (mg.)	Vitamin C (mg.)	Caloric Equivalents and Remarks
40	24	Good thiamine, riboflavin, niacin, B_6 and B_{12}	N/A*	Except for Pizza Supreme, one-half of a thin-crust pizza at Pizza Hut has fewer calories than a Big Mac, with comparable protein; ½ of a thick-crust pizza has from 20 to 100 more calories than thin-crust pizza. Except for scant vitamin C, these pizzas provide 25 to 40% of daily needs for nutrients listed.
N/A	N/A	N/A	N/A	
N/A	N/A	N/A	N/A	
N/A	N/A	N/A	N/A	
N/A	N/A	N/A	N/A	
50	30	Good thiamine, riboflavin, niacin, B_6 and B_{12}	8	
N/A	N/A	N/A	N/A	
N/A	N/A	N/A	N/A	
N/A	N/A	N/A	N/A	
N/A	N/A	N/A	N/A	
N/A	N/A	N/A	N/A	
0.3	160	Scant	4	½ orange; ⅓ apple. Compact size makes plums good snack item.

(continued)

FOOD RATING AND EVALUATION TABLE—*Continued*

Food	Portion	Calories	N/C Rating	Protein (g.)	Calcium (mg.)
Popcorn, buttered	2 cups	82	Poor	1.8	2
Pork					
Cured ham, lean and fat	6 oz.	490	Fair to good	36	16
Boiled ham (luncheon meat)	2 oz.	135	Fair to good	10	6
Chops, lean and fat	2 thick chops (3.5 oz. each)	520	Fair to very good (see Remarks)	32	16
Roast, lean and fat	6 oz.	620	Poor to very good (see Remarks)	42	18
Sausage	1 patty (2 oz. before cooking)	129	Poor	4.9	2

Food Rating and Evaluation Guide

Iron (mg.)	Vitamin A (I.U.)	B vitamins (mg.)	Vitamin C (mg.)	Caloric Equivalents and Remarks
0.4	0	Scant	0	½ large candy bar. If you can eat 1 or 2 cups and stop, not too bad a snack, supplying a little fiber and iron. But not much better than a brownie. Without butter, I'd rate it "fair."
4.4	0	Excellent	0	6 oz. pot roast, lean and fat; 7 oz. roasted chicken. Pork is obviously nutritious but tends to be fattier than beef or chicken. Trimmed of visible fat, it's much better.
1.6	0	Excellent	0	This is enough to make a sandwich, which would have 285 calories. With mayonnaise, about 335; with cheese, 385 or more.
4.4	0	Outstand-ing	0	These chops contain a total of only 4.6 oz. of meat, and of that 1.5 oz. is fat. Trim all fat off these chops and you'd have only 260 calories— a 50% reduction. And the calorie/protein ratio would be as good as lean ground beef.
5.4	0	Outstand-ing	0	The rating would jump to "Very good" if trimmed of fat—reducing fat from 28% to 14% and cutting calories to 350. In the same class as lean-only rib roast.
0.6	0	Good	0	A cooked sausage patty is 44% fat. You're much better off eating ham with your eggs. A small sausage link has 62 calories. 2 links, 2 eggs, 2 pieces buttered toast equals 568 calories.

(continued)

FOOD RATING AND EVALUATION TABLE—*Continued*

Food	Portion	Calories	N/C Rating	Protein (g.)	Calcium (mg.)
Potatoes					
Baked	1 large (2⅓″ × 4¾″)	145	Very good	4	14
French fries	10 strips (about 4″ long)	214	Poor	3.4	12
Mashed, milk and butter added	½ cup	99	Good	2.2	25
Chips	10	114	Poor	1.1	8
Potato salad, made with mayonnaise and eggs	½ cup	182	Fair	3.8	24
Pretzels	5 thin	117	Poor	3	7

Food Rating and Evaluation Guide

Iron (mg.)	Vitamin A (I.U.)	B vitamins (mg.)	Vitamin C (mg.)	Caloric Equivalents and Remarks
1.1	0	Excellent	31	Potatoes are practically fat-free, high in vitamins, minerals, and fiber. Learn to enjoy baked potatoes with small amount of butter or yogurt mashed in well. Also very high in potassium—3 times as much as an orange.
1	0	Good	16	A poor snack but not that bad a vegetable with dinner. Calorie for calorie, the nutritional profile is similar to apples. Fries from a restaurant, though, may have much less vitamin C, reducing rating to "Poor."
0.4	180	Good	10	½ cup beans or lentils. Surprisingly, has fewer calories than ½ cup applesauce and far more nutritive value. Go easy on the butter.
0.4	0	Scant	3	5 thin pretzels; ½ cup applesauce; 1 large brownie. These chips weigh less than an ounce. 2 ounces have 322 calories. Basically grease and salt, with some iron.
1	225	Good	14	1 cup coleslaw with mayonnaise; 3 oz. hamburger patty; 1 hot dog; 1 Devil Dog. It's the mayonnaise that dilutes a good food with empty calories.
0.45	0	Scant	0	14 almonds; 10 potato chips; 1 muffin; 2 oatmeal-raisin cookies. 1 Dutch pretzel has 62 calories. Thin pretzel sticks have 23 calories per 10 sticks and twice the salt of other pretzels.

(continued)

FOOD RATING AND EVALUATION TABLE–*Continued*

Food	Portion	Calories	N/C Rating	Protein (g.)	Calcium (mg.)
Prune juice	4 oz.	99	Fair to poor	0.5	18
Prunes ("softenized")	5 extra large	137	Fair to poor	1.2	27
Pudding					
Bread (with raisins)	½ cup	248	Fair to poor	7.4	145
Chocolate	½ cup	193	Poor	4.1	125
Rice, with raisins	½ cup	194	Fair to poor	4.8	130
Tapioca cream	½ cup	111	Fair to poor	4.2	87

Food Rating and Evaluation Guide

Iron (mg.)	Vitamin A (I.U.)	B vitamins (mg.)	Vitamin C (mg.)	Caloric Equivalents and Remarks
5.2 (outstand-ing)	0	Scant	3	NOTE: This is a 4-oz. glass, not 6. Higher in calories than other juices, it also has very low vitamin values, but very high iron value. Contains substance which stimulates bowels—unnaturally.
2.1 (excellent)	860	Good	2	⅓ cup dried apricots; 3 or 4 dried peach halves. Here's another basi-cally nutritious food that packs too many calories and is too conven-ient for snacking purposes. Would be rated "Good" for nonweight-conscious.
1.5	400	Good	2	1 small cup yogurt with sweetened fruit; 2 large slices Boston brown bread; 5 Oreos. A good dessert for those trying to gain weight.
7	195	Good riboflavin	1	½ cup rice pudding, to which it is similar except that it's completely lacking in fiber. Vanilla pudding, 142 calories, with slightly better nutritional profile.
0.6	145	Good riboflavin	0	Nutritious as desserts go, but that's a lot of calories for ½ cup—much more than ½ cup of ice cream (127).
0.4	240	Scant	1	Scant ½ cup ice cream; 1 large brownie; ¼ cup chocolate pudding. Won't win any nutrition prizes but calorie for calorie is better than 3 desserts mentioned.

(continued)

FOOD RATING AND EVALUATION TABLE—*Continued*

Food	Portion	Calories	N/C Rating	Protein (g.)	Calcium (mg.)
Pumpkin seeds	1 oz.	157	Good (in moderation)	8	14
Radishes	5 medium	4	Excellent	2.5	7
Raisins	⅓ cup (1½ oz.)	124	Poor	1.1	27
Rice					
Brown	½ cup	116	Very good	2.5	12
White ("enriched")	½ cup	112	Good	2.1	11

Food Rating and Evaluation Guide

Iron (mg.)	Vitamin A (I.U.)	B vitamins (mg.)	Vitamin C (mg.)	Caloric Equivalents and Remarks
3	20	Little	0	1 oz. sunflower seeds; 1 oz. cashews; 1 cup milk. Seeds are very concentrated sources of protein, iron, trace minerals—and oil. Another "health food" that has to be eaten with control to avoid caloric excess.
0.3	0	Scant	6	Calorie for calorie, one of the most efficient foods for delivering calcium, iron and vitamins. But because the amount we can eat is limited, only the vitamin C is significant.
1.5	15	Scant	0	The same number of calories in other dried fruits or nuts would give far more nutritive value. Iron here is good, though. A good snack for slender children. Adults can use as garnish.
0.5	0	Good	0	1 small baked potato; ½ cup beef and vegetable stew. Rice is best eaten as a "bed" for stews containing some lean meat and lots of vegetables. Brown rice is filling without being heavy.
0.9	0	Fair to good	0	Lacks fiber and some very important trace nutrients found in brown rice, but still a good food. Avoid eating drenched with butter.

(continued)

FOOD RATING AND EVALUATION TABLE—*Continued*

Food	Portion	Calories	N/C Rating	Protein (g.)	Calcium (mg.)
Rolls and buns					
Hard roll; e.g., Kaiser ("enriched")	1	156	Poor	4.9	24
Frankfurter or hamburger bun	1	119	Poor	3.3	30
Rye wafers	5	112	Fair to poor	4.3	17
Salad Dressings					
Commercial French	1 tsb.	66	Poor	0.1	2
Mayonnaise	1 tbs.	101	Poor	0.2	3
Salami	3 slices (about 1 oz.)	135	Poor	7.2	3

Food Rating and Evaluation Guide

Iron (mg.)	Vitamin A (I.U.)	B vitamins (mg.)	Vitamin C (mg.)	Caloric Equivalents and Remarks
1.2	0	Fair	0	2 pieces white bread. Lack of fiber and depletion of important trace nutrients makes any white bread product less than desirable. Rolls also invite use of lots of butter, sandwiches of fatty luncheon meat and mayonnaise.
0.8	0	Little	0	2 rolls with hot dogs equal 590 calories.
1.3	0	Fair	0	Better than white bread (these are whole grain wafers), but snacks should have fewer calories, more vitamins.
0.1	0	0	0	You can tell at a glance that adding more than 2 tbs. to a salad turns a low-calorie dish into a greasy orgy.
0.1	40	0	0	The most caloric salad dressing. All dressings are empty-calorie condiments differing only in calories per tablespoon—Blue, 76; Italian, 83; Russian, 74; Thousand Island, 80. Low-calorie dressings average about 25 calories per tbs. If you use 2 tbs. per salad, you save 100 calories.
1.2	0	Scant	0	2 oz. boiled ham (which has more protein and iron). Salami is 38% fat and contains undesirable additives.

(continued)

FOOD RATING AND EVALUATION TABLE—*Continued*

Food	Portion	Calories	N/C Rating	Protein (g.)	Calcium (mg.)
Salmon					
Sockeye, canned	3 oz.	145	Excellent	17.2	220 (if you eat the bone)
Baked, with butter	6 oz.	312	Excellent	46.2	0
Sardines	1 can (drained of oil)	187	Very good	22.1	402 (outstanding—comes from bones)
Sauerkraut	½ cup	21	Excellent	1.2	43
Scallops (breaded and fried)	6⅔ oz. (15 to 20 small)	367	Fair to poor	34	

*N/A = not available

Food Rating and Evaluation Guide

Iron (mg.)	Vitamin A (I.U.)	B vitamins (mg.)	Vitamin C (mg.)	Caloric Equivalents and Remarks
1	196	Outstand-ing	0	2½ oz. lean ground beef; 6 average sardines. What makes a salmon so much better than the salami above? Being a natural, unprocessed food, it has only 9% fat and isn't diluted by additives.
1.8 (excellent)	300	Excellent	0	7 oz. bluefish; 7 oz. fried chicken. Similar in value to lean beef, but with less iron. Smoked salmon (lox) has 50 calories per oz.
2.7 (excellent)	200	Good	0	The reason sardines aren't "Excellent" is because of their high salt content and the tendency to eat them with mayonnaise. If you don't drain the can of oil, you have 330 calories here.
0.6 (good)	60	Scant	17	Here's something you can fill yourself on, getting good vitamin C and iron in the process. Try kraut instead of potato salad.
See Remarks	N/A*	N/A	N/A	Scallops are similar to lobster in that they are practically fat-free and very high in protein—and also very expensive. The problem is the breading and frying—made far worse by dipping in tartar sauce. Mineral and vitamin values for fried scallops have not been determined, but they are probably high in iron. They're also naturally high in sodium (salt).

(continued)

FOOD RATING AND EVALUATION TABLE—*Continued*

Food	Portion	Calories	N/C Rating	Protein (g.)	Calcium (mg.)
Shrimp (french-fried)	3 oz.	192	Fair to poor	17.4	60
Soups					
Commercial chicken noodle	1 cup	62	Fair	3.4	10
Minestrone	1 cup	105	Very good	4.9	37
Vegetable beef	1 cup	78	Very good	5.1	12

Food Rating and Evaluation Guide

Iron (mg.)	Vitamin A (I.U.)	B vitamins (mg.)	Vitamin C (mg.)	Caloric Equivalents and Remarks
1.8	0	Some niacin	0	If you've a yen for shrimp, eat them in a shrimp cocktail and get away with half the calories shown here. Also, remember that fried shrimp are usually served with melted butter and french fries.
0.5	50	Little niacin	0	Won't win any nutrition contests but note that it contains almost 50 calories less than 1 scrambled egg and 100 calories less than a single pancake. Also, hot soups are more satisfying than calories might suggest.
1	2,350	Little	0	1 slice buttered bread (the soup has twice the protein and far more vitamin A).
0.7	2,700	Little	0	1 slice unbuttered bread; ½ baked potato; 2 bites of a hot dog on bun. Bargain caloric price for high vitamin A, iron. Soup, cottage cheese, fruit make well-balanced lunch. Other caloric values per cup of soup (all values for soup diluted with water per instructions; if milk is used, add 80 calories per cup): cream of asparagus, 65; beef bouillon, 19; beef noodle, 67; chicken consommé, 22; cream of chicken, 94; chicken gumbo, 55; chicken with rice, 48; chicken vegetable, 76; clam chowder (Manhattan), 81; cream of mushroom, 134; onion, 65; green pea, 130; split pea, 145; tomato, 88; turkey noodle, 79; vegetarian vegetable, 78.

(continued)

FOOD RATING AND EVALUATION TABLE—*Continued*

Food	Portion	Calories	N/C Rating	Protein (g.)	Calcium (mg.)
Sour cream	1 cup	495	Poor	7	268
	1 tbs.	25	Poor	Scant	14
Soybeans					
Cooked	½ cup	117	Excellent	9.9	66
Curd. See Tofu					
Spaghetti (with meatballs, tomato sauce, Parmesan cheese)	1 cup	332	Excellent	18.6	124
Spinach (cooked)	1 cup	41	Excellent	5.4	167 (but not utilizable)
Squash, summer (boiled)	1 cup (sliced)	25	Excellent	1.6	45
Syrups (table blend)	1 tbs.	60	Poor	0	9
Tangerine	1 large	46	Good	0.8	40

Food Rating and Evaluation Guide

Iron (mg.)	Vitamin A (I.U.)	B vitamins (mg.)	Vitamin C (mg.)	Caloric Equivalents and Remarks
0.1	1,820	Good riboflavin	2	Caloric murder as a dip base or on baked potatoes. Substituting yogurt, sour cream's twin, gives you one-fourth the calories and one-twelfth the fat for about the same amount of protein, calcium and B vitamins.
Scant	90	Scant	Scant	
2.5	25	Good	0	½ cup ordinary beans; 1 cup peas. Soybeans contain valuable nutrients, like lecithin, not shown on chart.
3.7	1,590	Excellent	22	2 slices pizza; 1 small hamburger on bun. High grades in all nutritional depts. Limit bread and eat without butter. A satisfying dish.
4 (usefulness limited)	14,580	Good	50	Traditionally valued for iron, the minerals here are largely unavailable. Best values are vitamins A and C—which are excellent. See Kale.
0.7	700	Some	18	Here's another garden vegetable you can eat your fill of. Mixes well with other vegetables and soups.
0.8	0	0	0	A good condiment for people with malnutrition and anemia—for all others, pure fat-power with a shot of iron. Avoid dishes that require syrup to be palatable.
0.4	420	Scant	31	⅔ orange; ½ apple or nectarine. Not quite as nutritious as oranges but better than apples. A decent snack but oranges may be safer—they're harder to peel.

(continued)

FOOD RATING AND EVALUATION TABLE−*Continued*

Food	Portion	Calories	N/C Rating	Protein (g.)	Calcium (mg.)
Tartar sauce	1 tbs.	74	Poor	0.2	3
Tofu (soybean curd)	1 piece (2½″ × 2¾″ × 1″)	86	Excellent	9.4	154
Tomato	1 (3″ dia.; 7 oz.)	40	Excellent	2	24
Tomato juice cocktail	1 glass (6 fl. oz.)	38	Very good	1.3	18
Toppings, whipped					
Cool Whip	1 tbs.	16	Poor	N/A*	N/A
Lucky Whip	1 tbs.	11	Poor	N/A	N/A
Snow-Kist	1 tbs.	15	Poor	N/A	N/A
D-Zerta (prepared from mix)	1 tbs.	7	Poor	N/A	N/A

*N/A = not available

Food Rating and Evaluation Guide

Iron (mg.)	Vitamin A (I.U.)	B vitamins (mg.)	Vitamin C (mg.)	Caloric Equivalents and Remarks
0.1	30	0	0	¾ tbs. mayonnaise; ½-plus tbs. oil. Another high-calorie, fatty condiment. Avoid foods you can't enjoy without it—they tend to be full of fat on their own—e.g., batter-fried fish sandwiches.
2.3	0	Scant	0	1 large egg; 1½ oz. flounder; 3 oz. cottage cheese; 1½ oz. lean hamburger. Good source of calcium and iron. Excellent nonmeat source of protein.
0.9	1,640	Fair	42	½ apple; 2 beets; 1 cup broccoli; 1 wedge cantaloupe. This is larger than prepackaged tomatoes, which are not worth eating anyway. Grow them yourself to get highest vitamin content and flavor.
1.6	1,460	Little	29	½ glass apple juice or orange juice. Much better than apple juice. Has less vitamin C than orange juice but much more iron and vitamin A. Only drawback is high sodium (salt) content. Add lemon juice and sip slowly for snack. Avoid at night; salt may cause sleeping problems.
N/A	N/A	N/A	N/A	Most whipped toppings are lower in calories than whipped cream itself (27 per tbs.), but still rate "Poor" nutritionally.
N/A	N/A	N/A	N/A	
N/A	N/A	N/A	N/A	
N/A	N/A	N/A	N/A	

(continued)

FOOD RATING AND EVALUATION TABLE—*Continued*

Food	Portion	Calories	N/C Rating	Protein (g.)	Calcium (mg.)
Toppings, whipped—*continued*					
Dream Whip (prepared from mix)	1 tbs.	14	Poor	N/A	N/A
Tuna					
Canned in oil; solids and liquid	1 can (6½ oz.; chunk style)	530	Fair	44.5	11
Same as above but drained of oil	1 can (same as above)	309	Excellent	45.2	13
Canned in water	1 can (same as above)	234	Excellent	51.5	29
Tuna salad	1 cup (7.3 oz.)	349	Fair	29.9	41

Iron (mg.)	Vitamin A (I.U.)	B vitamins (mg.)	Vitamin C (mg.)	Caloric Equivalents and Remarks
N/A	N/A	N/A	N/A	
2	170	Outstanding niacin	0	11 oz. broiled halibut; 6½ oz. ground beef. The halibut would give you twice the protein and a dozen times more A (if you could eat all 11 oz.). The beef is similar in value but has 6 times more iron. Canned tuna is very high in salt and oil. In fact, more than half the calories here are from the oil.
3	130	Outstanding niacin	0	6 oz. broiled halibut; 3 oz. regular ground beef. Note the caloric saving achieved by draining the oil. Adding 2 tbs. of mayonnaise would negate this saving. Tuna sandwich would have about half this much tuna.
2.9	0	Outstanding niacin	0	5 oz. broiled halibut; 3 oz. regular ground beef. Water-pack tuna has an extraordinary calorie/protein ratio of only 4.5, making it an unexcelled source of calorie-cheap protein. You'd have to eat 8 eggs (650 calories) to get all that protein.
2.7	590	Outstanding niacin	2	You can improve the rating to "Good" by going very light on the mayonnaise and adding extra tomato, onion, green peppers, carrots, bean sprouts. Celery adds bulk but no real nutrition.

(continued)

FOOD RATING AND EVALUATION TABLE—*Continued*

Food	Portion	Calories	N/C Rating	Protein (g.)	Calcium (mg.)
Turkey (roasted, white and dark meat)	6 oz. (6 small pieces)	324	Excellent	53.6	14
Turnips (cooked, cubed)	½ cup	18	Excellent	0.6	27
Veal					
Cutlet (medium fat)	6 oz.	370	Very good to excellent	46	18
Roast (medium fat)	6 oz.	460	Very good	46	20
Vegetable juice cocktail	1 glass (6 fl. oz.)	31	Excellent	1.6	22
Vegetables, mixed	½ cup	58	Excellent	2.9	23

Food Rating and Evaluation Guide

Iron (mg.)	Vitamin A (I.U.)	B vitamins (mg.)	Vitamin C (mg.)	Caloric Equivalents and Remarks
3	0	Excellent niacin	0	Similar to chicken and lean beef. Avoid eating large portions of skin and making sandwiches with lots of mayonnaise. Use tomato to moisten. Sandwich with 3 oz. meat, whole wheat bread, 1 tsp. mayonnaise has about 325 calories—not bad.
0.3	0	Scant	17	Here's a good starchy food you can fill up on as long as you go easy on the butter. Use cooking liquid to provide moisture instead. Who said starchy foods are fattening?
5.4	0	Very good	0	6½ oz. lean pot roast; 7 oz. white meat chicken; 8 oz. broiled bluefish. Veal has an excellent calorie/protein ratio, and the iron in veal is especially well utilized.
5.8	0	Excellent	0	6 oz. lean and fat broiled round. You can see that veal roast is fattier than cutlets. While highly nutritious, here is a food that you can easily eat too much of.
0.9	1,270	Some niacin	16	One of the few recreational beverages that doesn't contain lots of empty calories. Try adding lemon and spices for a good snack. Only drawback is high sodium content.
1.2	4,505	Fair	8	⅓ large baked potato; ½ cup peas. Try eating a smaller meat portion and a whole cup of mixed vegetables tossed with a small amount of butter. Good vitamin A, iron.

(continued)

FOOD RATING AND EVALUATION TABLE—*Continued*

Food	Portion	Calories	N/C Rating	Protein (g.)	Calcium (mg.)
Waffle (baked from mix, using egg and milk)	1 (7″ dia.)	206	Poor	6.6	179
Walnuts, English	1 oz. (about 14 small halves)	185	Poor	4.2	28
Watercress	1 cup	7	Excellent	0.8	53
Watermelon	1 large wedge (4″ thick, 8″ radius)	111	Excellent	2.1	30
Wheat germ (toasted, no added sugar)	6 tbs.	138	Excellent	11	18
Yeast, brewer's	1 tbs.	23	Outstanding	3.1	17

Food Rating and Evaluation Guide

Iron (mg.)	Vitamin A (I.U.)	B vitamins (mg.)	Vitamin C (mg.)	Caloric Equivalents and Remarks
1	170	Fair	. 0	2 scrambled eggs (which would give twice the protein); ¾ container fruit yogurt (giving 50% more calcium and two-thirds more protein). The worst thing about waffles is this: 1 waffle plus 2 pats of butter plus 3 tbs. syrup equals 455 calories. You might as well eat a steak.
0.9	10	Little	1	2 dozen almonds; 3 peaches. All nuts are nutritious and contain minerals not listed here—but the nourishment comes at too high a caloric price.
0.6	1,720	Scant	28	Another virtually calorie-free salad green, high in vitamins.
2.1	2,510	Fair	30	½ cup applesauce; 1 large banana; ¾ cantaloupe; 2 peaches. A good snack, rich in vitamins and potassium. If you have a tendency to overdo watermelon, cantaloupe may be more filling.
2.5	60	Excellent	6	1 large cup oatmeal; 1 jumbo scrambled egg; 1 thick slice toast with butter and jelly. Wheat germ is one health food that deserves its reputation. Especially valuable for B vitamins, iron, fiber and trace nutrients.
1.4	0	Outstanding	0	Another special food—of special interest to the weight-conscious because it contains Glucose Tolerance Factor, which improves metabolism of sugar and tends to lower high levels of insulin (common in heavy people), and possibly decreases too-keen appetite.

(continued)

FOOD RATING AND EVALUATION TABLE—*Continued*

Food	Portion	Calories	N/C Rating	Protein (g.)	Calcium (mg.)
Yogurt, plain (made with partially skim milk)	8 oz. (1 container)	113	Excellent	7.7	271

SOURCES: Adapted from
Agriculture Handbook Nos. 8 and 456 (Washington, D.C.: U.S. Department of Agriculture).
"Body Weight-Gain Equivalents of Selected Foods," by Frank Konishi and Sharon L. Harrison, *Journal of the American Dietetic Association,* 1977.
Brand Name Guide to Calories and Carbohydrates, by William I. Kaufman (New York: Pyramid Books, 1973).
Calories and Carbohydrates, by Barbara Kraus (New York: Grosset and Dunlap, 1971).
"Fast Food: Where's the Nutrition," by Marion J. Franz, in *Diabetes Forecast,* American Diabetes Association, 1985.

Food Rating and Evaluation Guide

Iron (mg.)	Vitamin A (I.U.)	B vitamins (mg.)	Vitamin C (mg.)	Caloric Equivalents and Remarks
0.1	150	High in riboflavin	2	1 glass (6 fl. oz.) milk; 1 oz. cheddar cheese. Note this is plain yogurt-flavored yogurt may have 240–280 calories, the difference a result of added sugar. Try combining plain with wheat germ and fresh fruit for complete nutrition.

"Fast Food and the American Diet," American Council on Science and Health, September, 1985.
Home and Garden Bulletin No. 72 (Washington, D.C.: U.S. Department of Agriculture).
"Nutritional Analysis of Food Served at McDonald's Restaurants," by WARF Institute, Inc. (Oak Brook, Ill.: McDonald's System, 1977).
"Nutritional Information Chart" Pizza Hut, Inc., April 1977.

NOTE: All meat values are for cooked meat.

Index

Page numbers for entries in tables appear in *italics*.

A

Abdomen
    exercise for, 84
    poor muscle tone in, 81
Acidosis, 117
Acne, cleared up by zinc, 182
Activities, common daily, calo-
    ries burned by, 233-37,
    236-49
Aging, 195-96
Alcohol, 132-33, 209-10. *See
    also* Beer; Liquor, hard;
    Wine
Almonds, 158, *258-59*
Amaranth, *160-61, 258-59*

Anemia
    from dieting, 117
    from folate deficiency, 118
    iron deficiency, 118, 175
Anorexia, 88
Appetite. *See also* Eating; Hunger
    reduced by exercise, 79
    reduced by water, 221
    suppressed by ketone
        bodies, 197
Appetite control system, 47-48
Apples, *258-59*
    baked, 149
Apple juice, *174, 260-61*
Applesauce, *260-61*
Apricot nectar, *260-61*

351

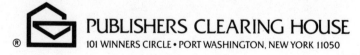